BIRD FLU

A Rising Pandemic in Asia and Beyond?

BIRD FLU

A Rising Pandemic in Asia and Beyond?

Paul TAMBYAH

National University of Singapore

Ping-Chung LEUNG

Chinese University of Hong Kong

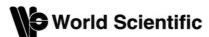

World Scientific

NEW JERSEY · LONDON · SINGAPORE · BEIJING · SHANGHAI · HONG KONG · TAIPEI · CHENNAI

Published by

World Scientific Publishing Co. Pte. Ltd.

5 Toh Tuck Link, Singapore 596224

USA office: 27 Warren Street, Suite 401-402, Hackensack, NJ 07601

UK office: 57 Shelton Street, Covent Garden, London WC2H 9HE

British Library Cataloguing-in-Publication Data
A catalogue record for this book is available from the British Library.

BIRD FLU
A Rising Pandemic in Asia and Beyond?

Copyright © 2006 by World Scientific Publishing Co. Pte. Ltd.

ISBN   981-256-815-8
ISBN   981-256-807-7 (pbk)

Typeset by Stallion Press
Email: enquiries@stallionpress.com

Printed in Singapore by Mainland Press

Contents

Contributors

Nugroho Abikusno
Associate Professor in Public Health
    and Medical Nutrition
Center for Community Health
    and Population Studies
Faculty of Medicine
Trisakti University
Jakarta, Indonesia

Anucha Apisarnthanarak
Division of Infectious Diseases
Faculty of Medicine
Thammasart University Hospital
Pratumthani, Thailand

Louis Y.-A. Chai
Registrar
Department of Medicine
National University Hospital
Singapore

Paul K.-S. Chan
Professor
Department of Microbiology
The Chinese University of Hong Kong
Prince of Wales Hospital
Hong Kong SAR, China

Vincent T.-K. Chow
Associate Professor
Department of Microbiology
Yong Loo Lin School of Medicine
National University of Singapore

Salin Chutinimitkul
Center of Excellence in Viral Hepatitis Research
Department of Pediatrics
Faculty of Medicine
Chulalongkorn University
Bangkok, Thailand

Dale A. Fisher
Associate Professor
Department of Medicine
Yong Loo Lin School of Medicine
National University of Singapore

Raymond Gani
Microbial Risk Assessment
Centre for Emergency Preparedness and Response
Health Protection Agency
Salisbury, Wiltshire, UK

I Nyoman Kandun
Director General
Directorate General for Disease
    Control and Environmental Health
Ministry of Health
Government of Indonesia

Thana Khawcharoenporn
Division of Infectious Diseases
Faculty of Medicine
Thammasart University Hospital
Pratumthani, Thailand

David S.-Q. Koh
Professor and Head
Department of Community, Occupational
    and Family Medicine
Yong Loo Lin School of Medicine
National University of Singapore

Gerald C.-H. Koh
Assistant Professor
Department of Community, Occupational
    and Family Medicine
Yong Loo Lin School of Medicine
National University of Singapore

Richard M. Krause
Senior Investigator
National Institute of Allergy and Infectious Diseases
    and Senior Scientific Advisor
Fogarty International Center
National Institutes of Health
Maryland, USA

Ronald M.-K. Lam
Principal Medical and Health Officer
Emergency Response and Information Branch
Centre for Health Protection
Department of Health
Hong Kong SAR, China

Vernon J. Lee
Public Health Registrar
Department of Clinical Epidemiology
Communicable Disease Centre
Tan Tock Seng Hospital
Singapore

Pak-Yin Leung
Controller
Centre for Health Protection
Department of Health
Hong Kong SAR, China

Ping-Chung Leung
Chairman, Management Committee
Centre for Clinical Trials on Chinese Medicine
The Institute of Chinese Medicine (ICM)
The Chinese University of Hong Kong
Hong Kong SAR, China

Nuning M.K. Masjkuri
Epidemiology Department
Faculty of Public Health
University of Indonesia
Depok, Indonesia

Linda M. Mundy
Saint Louis University School of Public Health
Saint Louis, MO, USA

Kai-Hong Phua
Joint Associate Professor
Department of Community, Occupational
   and Family Medicine
Yong Loo Lin School of Medicine
   and the Lee Kuan Yew School of Public Policy
National University of Singapore

Yong Poovorawan
Center of Excellence in Viral Hepatitis Research
Department of Pediatrics
Faculty of Medicine
Chulalongkorn University
Bangkok, Thailand

Pattaratida Sa-nguanmoo
Center of Excellence in Viral Hepatitis Research
Department of Pediatrics
Faculty of Medicine
Chulalongkorn University
Bangkok, Thailand

Hari Santoso
Chief of Outbreaks Control
Surveillance Subdirectorate
Directorate General for Disease
    Control and Environmental Health
Ministry of Health
Government of Indonesia

Rita Y.-T. Sung
Professor
Department of Paediatrics
The Chinese University of Hong Kong
Prince of Wales Hospital
Hong Kong SAR, China

Paul A. Tambyah
Associate Professor and Head
Infectious Diseases Section
Department of Medicine
Yong Loo Lin School of Medicine
National University of Singapore

Tri Yunis Miko Wahyono
Epidemiology Department
Faculty of Public Health
University of Indonesia
Depok, Indonesia

Glossary

Vocabulary	Definition
Antibiotic	A medication used to treat bacterial infections.
Antibody	A protein produced by the body's immune system that recognizes and helps fight infections and other foreign substances in the body.
Antigenic	An antigen is a molecule that stimulates the production of antibodies. Usually, it is a protein or a polysaccharide, from some external substance including an infection.
Asymptomatic infection	An infection which does not produce any symptoms at all. In other words, a silent infection.
Autopsy	A surgical procedure after death which involves the examination of body tissues, often to determine cause of death.
Bacteremia	Presence of bacteria in the blood.
Cardiac dilatation	Swelling of the heart.
Conjunctival	The white part of the eye.
Creatinine	A waste substance produced by the body usually cleared by the kidneys. It rises in concentration when the kidneys are not working.
Cytopathic effect	Something (usually a virus) that causes cells usually in a laboratory to be damaged or to die.
Dyspnea	Shortness of breath, difficult or labored breathing.
Encephalitis	A condition characterized by inflammation of the brain.
Encephalopathy	Disease of the brain.
Epidemiological	A branch of medical science that deals with the incidence, distribution, and control of disease in a population.
Epistaxis	Nose bleeding.
Erythrocyte	Red blood cell; contains hemoglobin, which carries oxygen to the tissues.

Vocabulary	Definition
Fluorescein	A fluorescent molecule which, after absorbing light, excites an electron and emits fluorescent light which is used to detect certain reactions in laboratories.
Genetic reassortment	Mixing of the genes — this can include genes from the same virus or bacteria or different organisms.
Genotype	The specific genetic makeup of an individual, usually in the form of DNA. It codes for the phenotype (or characteristics) of that individual.
Glycoprotein	A molecule that is composed of a protein molecule linked to a carbohydrate molecule.
Haemagglutination	The agglutination or clumping of red blood cells by virus.
Haemagglutinin	An antigenic glycoprotein found on the surface of the Influenza virus and is responsible for binding the virus to the cell that is being infected.
Horizontal transmission	Contagion or spread of an infectious disease from one individual to another within a population, independent of the parental relationship of those individuals. Contrast with vertical transmission.
Hyperglycemia	High blood sugar.
Immunofluorescence	The use of a fluorescent marker molecule to demonstrate linkage to a specific antibody. This is used to detect the presence of antibodies in laboratories.
Immunological	Anything that pertains to the body's natural defenses or immunity against disease.
Influenza prophylaxis	Prevention of influenza.
Inhalation	Taking a substance, typically in the form of gases, fumes, vapors, mists, aerosols or dusts, into the body by breathing it in.
Interferon	An antiviral substance produced by the body. It can also be synthesized.
Interleukin	A chemical substance that is produced by the body usually in response to inflammation.
Intranasal	In the nose.
Leucopenia	A decrease in the number of circulating white cells in the blood.
Lymphopenia	The condition in which there exists an abnormally low number of lymphocytes, a type of white blood cell, in the blood.
Malaise	Tiredness.
Matrix protein	A structural protein playing a role in the assembly of the virus particle.

Vocabulary	Definition
Monoclonal antibody	An antibody (a type of protein) designed by scientists to target one kind of cell. Monoclonal antibodies may be made of mouse proteins, by combining human and mouse proteins, or by using only human proteins.
Mortality	The rate of death.
Myalgia	Muscle ache.
Neuraminidase	An important surface structure protein of the influenza virus, an essential enzyme for the spread of the virus throughout the respiratory tract, enables the virus to escape the host cell and infect new cells.
Nucleoprotein	Conjugated protein composed of nucleic acid and protein; the material of which the chromosomes are made.
Oropharyngeal swab	Taking of mucus in throat by using a small piece of material, such as gauze or cotton.
Parenchyma	The tissue of an organ (as distinguished from supporting or connective tissue).
PCR	Polymerase Chain Reaction, a technique that uses an enzyme (DNA polymerase) to repeatedly amplify specific regions of a DNA molecule, as a result of cycles of denaturation, polymerization and elongation.
Pneumothorax	Air in the space outside the lungs. This is a disease condition as air is supposed to be inside the lungs not outside it.
Polymorphism	Difference in DNA sequence among individuals. Genetic variations occurring in more than 1% of a population would be considered useful polymorphisms for genetic linkage analysis.
Pulmonary hemorrhage	Bleeding in the lungs.
Radiographic	Using X-rays.
Rhinitis	Running nose.
RT-PCR	Real Time PCR. A method of doing the polymerase chain reaction in a more compact and rapid way.
Sepsis syndrome	A syndrome characterized by a rapid heart rate or breathing rate, abnormally high or low temperature, abnormally high or low white blood cell counts and the presence of infection.
Serological	A medical blood test to detect the presence of antibodies against a microorganism.
Seropositivity	Positive results from a serological test.

Vocabulary	Definition
Severe respiratory disease	Severe disease related to organs that are involved in breathing. These include the nose, throat, larynx, trachea, bronchi, and lungs.
Sputum	Mucus and other matter that is brought up from the lungs by coughing.
Supraventricular tachyarrhythmia	An abnormal heart rhythm that can result from damage to the atrium, lungs or changes in blood chemistry among other causes.
Syndrome	A set of symptoms or conditions that occur together and suggest the presence of a certain disease or an increased chance of developing the disease.
Thrombocytopenia	A decrease in the number of platelets in the blood.
Transaminase	An enzyme present in the liver.
Trivalent influenza vaccine	An influenza vaccine that protects against three different strains of influenza.
Tumor necrosis factor-alpha	A chemical mediator produced by the body as part of the inflammatory response.
Vertical transmission	Transfer of a pathogen from a parent to the offspring through reproduction.
Viremia	Presence of virus in the blood.

Foreword

We live in an amazing time in influenza. The H5N1 "bird flu" virus has spread from its epicenter in southern China, and is being tracked in avian hosts in eastern Asia to focal points across the Eurasian land mass to northern Africa. Although widespread in occurrence, it remains to be seen whether it will give rise to a pandemic. Regardless of outcome, this event marks a remarkable turning point in history — the world has, for the first time, a warning of a possible pandemic and a tangible one at that. Nine years on since the initial recognition of the H5N1 virus in chicken and a child in Hong Kong, the H5N1 saga continues. The virus is proving a formidable quarry, as its spread is registered, action taken and its genetic and antigenic features determined seeking signs indicative of changes in human pathogenicity and transmissibility.

The key to dealing with these issues lies in influenza virus surveillance, ideally knowing what viruses occur normally in animals and birds, particularly domestic poultry and wild birds, so that when a suspect virus appears authorities can react positively and confidently at the baseline avian level. To do so requires long term political will and support. Hong Kong has effectively functioned as an influenza sentinel post for many years. Virus surveillance in the aftermath of the 1997 H5N1 outbreak detected H5N1 activity in poultry in 1999 from southern China, the recognition of a number of H5N1 genotypes by 2002 including a dominant genotype designated Z. It was this genotype that predominated in the "bird flu" outbreak in eastern Asia, particularly southeast Asia, when the virus's presence was made known in late 2003–2004 and voyages that have since followed. The "bird flu" virus cauldron still bubbles in southern China and parts of southeast Asia and it now threatens in points beyond.

It is timely to take stock of the experience of those in the wider region in dealing with the disease in humans and at the avian level. Those involved with the "bird flu" are fully occupied with the many issues that the H5N1 virus has presented. This compendium provides a glimpse of them which may be of benefit to those near and afar. It draws upon new faces in the influenza arena, especially so as they and many others grapple with the virus.

In a number of ways, the saga has brought together many people who are contributing for the common good, not only in those areas affected by the virus, but parties from around the world who have, through their governments and agencies, contributed manpower to the "H5N1 war effort." These people will be able to take their experiences back to their home countries for better preparedness and action should the need arise.

In its "early" days, the present H5N1 virus was promiscuous, i.e. reassorting its genes with abandon with other avian influenza viruses, leading to the emergence of the dominant Z genotype. It might be considered to be now in a "smouldering" phase, a phase that may have preceded the catastrophic 1918 pandemic in its most likely source in southern China, waiting for the right genetic event to trigger it into pandemicity either through tweaking its own machinery possibly in terrestrial poultry, or through genetic reconfiguration resulting from reassortment with one or other influenza viruses. In the case of the latter, resulting reassortant progeny viruses may or may not maintain subtype H5N1 virus antigenicity. The importance of virus surveillance and genetic examination of all avian influenza virus isolates additional to H5N1 isolates cannot be over-stressed, full well appreciating the difficulties and greater burden these entail.

Thus, important as H5N1 is, investigators must keep a watchful eye for other influenza viruses entering the H5N1 equation or usurping it. All the more so, since it has now entered an insidious phase living for the most part asymptomatically in domestic ducks in the region, a phase that its "sister" H9N2 virus seemingly did a few years earlier. This phase facilitates a greater opportunity long-term for the H5N1 virus to reassort with, say, H9N2 or H4N6, the most common virus subtype in domestic ducks, with consequences unknown. As background to this, the H3 subtype is, or at least was, the second most frequent virus H subtype in ducks and it gave rise to the H3N2 pandemic virus of 1968 in southern China possibly facilitated through the domestic pig as a virus "mixing vessel." It has been my long held view on pandemic influenza to "expect the unexpected." Time is of the essence — in fact, effort must be redoubled. Additional dedicated manpower is of the order.

At a recent international forum in Beijing, around US$2 billion was pledged toward grappling the "bird flu" problem not only as a current threat to human health but also as a potential long-term threat through global spread and endemicity in avian hosts. This threat includes poultry — our principal meat protein source — as well as other avian hosts posing a direct threat to ecosystems. Asia stands to be a major beneficiary and it is important that core factors are addressed. It is critical that sound education in influenza reaches the appropriate people at all levels of government, and that those involved in the industry and poultry as a livelihood are made aware of the disease and its implications. Inculcation of the broader aspects of biosecurity are of paramount importance. These have ramifications for teaching in schools as well as university veterinary and biological sciences curricula. They also signal how little is really known about the ecology of influenza viruses. The time has come to reconsider animal farming practices generally, not only in the light of pandemic influenza but also others such as the severe acute respiratory syndrome (SARS) and bovine spongiform encephalopathy (BSE). Storm clouds are gathering for the emergence of newer and perhaps equally as dangerous zoonotic diseases.

These are uncertain influenza times, busy times, and the efforts of the contributors to this compendium are to be applauded, with the hope that many others will be able to draw upon it for the good of all — humans, animals and the well-being of the planet.

Kennedy F. Shortridge
Emeritus Professor, University of Hong Kong
9 March 2006

Preface

Whilst still recovering from the severe acute respiratory syndrome (SARS) disaster, another viral attack rears its ugly head. This one expected to be of much a bigger scale with more serious consequences — the Avian Flu Pandemic.

At our hospital where the SARS epidemic started two and a half years ago, wounds are still being repaired and regulations and rules for the repetition of high risk infections are still being laid down. Practical drills which should have been enjoyable off-work exercises have turned into preparatory lessons. In-service short training courses which flourished after the SARS crisis under the auspices of tertiary institutions and professional bodies, directed towards infection control, safety and health protections, suddenly appear untimely and overdue.

The Pandemic may come, sooner or later.
The Pandemic will come, any day.
Such are the believes and assumptions. Preparations need to be immediate.
From an academic viewpoint, do we support the assumption?

There are good reasons supporting those who believe that the pandemic will come. Firstly, there appear to be epidemic cycles with influenza infection. Virologists take 30 to 40 years as a probable peaceful period, beyond which an up-flare of influenza infections, amounting to an epidemic, would occur. The last worldwide flu epidemic occurred 37 years ago, originating in Asia. Hence, it is not without good reasoning and logic to speculate that Asia is expecting another new flu epidemic cycle to occur any time.

The threat appears particularly real since the H5N1 virus is a new strain that has been so virulent to birds and has already attacked humans. The new strain has not yet initiated the effective natural immunological defense yet, and therefore, will be particularly powerful for the creation of an epidemic, and pandemic.

Indeed the H5N1 strain has already demonstrated its utmost lethality: infected birds are probably suffering a 100% mortality; whereas infected humans demonstrated an average mortality of 50%. The more virulent the biological agent, the more capable it will be in initiating a widespread infection. Basing on the available data so far, the viral strain appears to be more virulent than any ever reported. The mortality rate during the 1918 Spanish pandemic, was taken to be only 5% in spite of the huge population affected; and even the SARS epidemic resulted in only a 10% mortality.

There are other observations supporting the assumption that the H5N1 pandemic will arrive in the near future.

If a biological agent infects through multiple channels, it will be more capable of initiating a pandemic. Indeed H5N1 has been found in respiratory secretions as well as in bowel excretions. Prevention of cross-infection therefore becomes more difficult.

In fact, the nature of the flu virus itself has been supportive of easy spread, unlike other viral infections. When the human individual catches the flu viral infection, he remains asymptomatic for about a week before there are symptom manifestations. If this individual moves around, he forms a good source of infection. With the increasing ease of modern travel, one can imagine the danger of such an infected and yet apparently healthy individual.

The past episodes of influenza epidemic were all related to the occurrence of new strains of the flu virus. New strains appear when old strains are allowed to reassort in different animals. Since H5N1 strains were found in birds, humans and even pigs, we are now reaching a really dangerous era of creating new virulent strains. The recent discovery that the 1918 virus responsible for the Spanish flu pandemic actually possessed DNA of bird origin added more weight to the threat.

One wishes that vaccines could be developed to counteract the impending epidemic. Nevertheless, the development of vaccine takes time. Moreover, creating potent vaccines for an ever mutating virus will be of utmost difficulty.

Not only is vaccination deficient, but treatment for the expected epidemic is equally problematic. Available drugs may be good for the conventional influenza infection, but with an unknown new strain there is no guarantee for their efficacy. Indeed some of the recently infected H5N1 patients were treated with anti-flu therapy which eventually failed to save their lives.

The likely occurrence of bird flu pandemic in Asia further sets a pessimistic scene. Large areas of Asia are still underdeveloped and backward. Control of infection spread will be particularly difficult in the poverty areas.

In spite of the pessimistic popular thinking, there are still optimists who disagree and are able to make observations of opposite view, i.e. even if bird flu becomes a reality, an epidemic outcome should not be disastrous. They think that:

(1) H5N1 epidemic may be just another flu episode, the imaginary disastrous results are all simple assumptions.
(2) Many people have had anti-flu vaccinations in the past and although the resulting immuno-modulating effects are not specific against bird flu, they must be helpful to different levels.
(3) We expect a gradual decline of virulence with viral infections that repeatedly infects individual animals and humans.
(4) Advances in public health and medicine have made our world today very different from in 1918; it is much more capable of fighting against epidemics. For example, means of isolation are much more adequate today.

Indeed, ever since an epidemic of infection has become known to human beings, isolation has been the most effective method of control of infection spread. Hong Kong did so badly during the SARS crises, because isolation had not been taken seriously and decisively. Rather, the health authorities were very proud of their hospital facilities and high quality manpower, capable of providing the most up-to-date treatment. The result of this specific confidence co-existing with the lack of broad general views of risk management and a deficient understanding of history, resulted in the uncontrolled community spread of infection. On the other hand, in Beijing, once the awareness of the infection getting out of control was firmly established, drastic measures to achieve isolation, both in the community and in the hospital, were administered. The dramatic set-up of the "little Chang-shan" hospital to accommodate all the infected patients was a perfect demonstration of the value of isolation in epidemic control. If the expected avian flu epidemic does not call for preparations for effective isolations, one worries that the SARS disaster will just repeat itself.

If infected poultry can be isolated, instead of being killed, as a means of controlling the spread of avian flu among poultry, perhaps the current threat may not be so real and worrying. When infected birds are just killed, we leave no chance for them to develop their natural defense against the invading virus. If they are not killed, the natural ecological order will protect the birds from extinction when the birds' defense system will be strengthened to fight against the virus. The downgrading virus then may not infect humans. Nevertheless, the wealth and complexity of the present global economical structure demands immediate results; keeping the poultry alive, isolating them and allowing Nature to maintain its balance have already become impossible.

Now that we are facing this real threat from avian flu, the chapter authors of this book intend to make the general public aware of it. Instead of developing a feeling of uncertainty and pessimism, they should be informed of what is really happening: from historical facts, viral infections, the current situation, vaccination, treatment, preparations against the expected epidemic, ecological considerations and the expected impacts of the epidemic. The book is designed for lay reading but the contents will have clear professional and scientific orientations.

Professor Ping-Chung Leung
Editor

A Summary of Flu Attacks

1890 The first clear historical record of an influenza epidemic.

1918 "The Spanish Influenza," starting in Europe, then America, and finally spreading all over the world. An estimated 40 to 60 million people died. The virus was found to be H1N1. Theory of virus origin is that of bird-bovine-human.

1957 The Asian Flu. Started in Asia, over 100,000 died, and the virus was H2N2.

1968 The Hong Kong Flu. Started in Hong Kong, spreading worldwide. Over 700,000 died. The virus was H3N2. Theory of viral origin: interchange of DNA between bird and human flu, i.e. same human individual infected with both viruses.

1997 The Hong Kong Bird Flu. Avian flu virus H5N1 isolated for the first time from an infected child; 18 infected, six died. All victims showed a strong history of close contact with birds.

2001 The World Health Organization (WHO) established the World Wide Surveillance System for influenza infection.

2003 The Avian Flu affected 800 chicken farms in Holland. Over 10 million chickens were slaughtered. Eighty-three persons were infected, one died. Virus was H7N7. Hong Kong had two people infected, one died. Korea caught the flu. Virus was H5N1.

2004 The Avian Flu started in Japan. Thailand and Vietnam caught the flu; infected 11 people, eight died. All of Southeast Asia was infected with the flu. Over 100 million chickens and ducks were slaughtered. The virus was N5N1.

2005 Vietnam, Cambodia, Indonesia and Korea reported Avian Flu outbreaks. Fifty million chickens and ducks were slaughtered. Mortality was high among infected humans: 12 out of 13 in Vietnam and one out of one in Cambodia. H5N1 was the virus responsible. Indonesia identified H5N1 in pigs. Later in the year, more countries declared the incidence of bird deaths because of H5N1. These countries included Russia, Romania, Turkey, Ukraine and Sandi Arabia. More mortalities were reported in Indonesia and Vietnam. The flu spread widely throughout many provinces in China with a few human infections.

2006 At the beginning of 2006, more than ten proven cases of Avian Flu were reported in different provinces of China and the mortality reached 40%–50%. The incidence appeared to be rising.
From February 2006 onwards, more H5N1-infected birds appeared in Greece, Italy, Austria, Croatia and Germany.

1

Avian Influenza: Basic Science, Potential for Mutation, Transmission, Illness Symptomatology and Vaccines

Louis Y.-A. Chai

Understanding the Basic Science of Influenza and Terminology

Influenza viruses belong to the family of viruses called *Orthomyxoviruses* ("myxo" meaning affinity for mucin) and are classified into three different types: influenza A, influenza B and influenza C. Most of the major historic pandemics to date have been ascribed to the former. Influenza A can be perceived as a roughly minute spherical particle with a size of approximately 80–120 nanometers, protected by an outer shell which radiates projecting spikes consisting of viral hemagglutinin and neuraminidase. Within the shell are eight single strands of genetic RNA material and additional viral non-structural (NS) proteins. The RNA codes for the specific character of the strain as determined by the respective hemagglutinin and neuraminidase components (Figure 1).

1

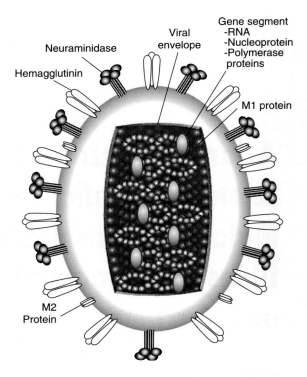

Figure 1: Schematic model of influenza virus.

The hemagglutinin (HA) and neuraminidase (NA) surface spikes are made of a sugar-protein structural concoction which combine to give individual influenza strains identity and aid in their disease-causing propensity through recognition and destruction of human cells. The main circulating HA and NA subtypes in humans currently are H1N1 and H3N2, respectively. In aquatic birds, all the different variations of the H and N occur naturally without causing disease. Thus ducks and geese can have various combinations of H1 to H16 and N1 to N9. Thus the variations in the H and N give rise to the names of various influenza strains like the H1N1 (responsible for the 1918 Spanish influenza pandemic) and H2N2 Asian pandemic strain of 1958–59.

Like all living organisms, influenza viruses are also subject to the process of natural selection, and undergo spontaneous genetic variation involving their HA and NA components. Depending on whether the variation is small or big, this is referred to as either **antigenic drift** or **antigenic shift**, respectively. Antigenic drift occurs when small changes occur but the H-type remains the same. For example, every year, there is antigenic drift and the

H1N1 circulating this year is slightly different from the H1N1 circulating last year, hence the need to get vaccinated every year against the different strains of the virus that are circulating. The same happens for the H3N2 which is circulating every year. On the other hand, if there is an antigenic shift, then instead of H1N1 and H3N2 circulating among humans, some novel strain such as H1-16N1-9 might suddenly emerge. This guise on the surface of the virus is one which the human immune system may not recognize as familiar, hence presenting a major health risk even to those who have had previous influenza attacks and would have attained some immunity to that infective strain. Influenza pandemics in history have largely resulted due to antigenic shifts with consequent phenomenal human-to-human spread due to host susceptibility to new influenza hemagglutinin strains such as H1N1 in 1918, H2N2 in 1957 and H3N2 in 1968.

Influenza Pandemics in Recent History

A pandemic signals a global outbreak of disease that occurs when a new influenza virus appears or emerges causing serious illness with high trans-missibility rates from person to person. This is in contrast to an epidemic which is defined as an outbreak of influenza confined to one location, for instance, a city, town or country. Almost all pandemics in recent history to date are caused by the human influenza A virus. This usually occurs with a new potent influenza A strain which arises as a result of antigenic shift and consequently is able to effectively infect a susceptible population.

The Great Pandemic of 1918–19, named the "Spanish Flu" was caused by an influenza A H1N1 strain swept past North America and Europe caus-ing an estimated 20–40 million deaths in the pre-antimicrobial era afflicting especially young working-age adults. Average national life expectancy in the United States during that dark period dropped from excess of 50 years old to less than 40 years old. This was followed by the "Asian Flu" pandemic which possibly emerged in spring 1957 in China of the H2N2 subtype which eventually reached the North American continent. In 1967–68, the "Hong Kong" pandemic was caused by H3N2, and since the late 1970s H1N1 and H3N2 subtypes of the influenza A virus have been co-circulating worldwide, which forms the basis of the trivalent influenza vaccine.

As can be seen, based on history, pandemics are projected to occur once every 10 to 30 years. The pandemic-causing strains are "new" to the immune system for which the population has minimal immunity and antibody pro-tection, hence the propensity to cause maximal disease. With each subse-quent "wave" of the same viral infection with time, the population gradually attains a "herd immunity" in the above time frame before natural conditions become right again for the cyclical emergence of a new influenza A strain, HxNy. As would have thus noted, the next great pandemic is notably far overdue.

Basic Science of Avian Influenza

Corresponding strains of influenza A can afflict animals like swine, horse, marine mammals and also birds. For instance ducks, geese, chicken (avian) influenza strains comprise of a varied permutation consisting of H1–15 and N1–9 subtypes, while influenza strains in pigs harbor H1, H3, N1, N2 and N7 subtypes. Avian influenza is certainly no novel emerging entity — the ailment has been known to afflict wild fowl and poultry since the turn of the 20th century causing morbidty/mortality in wild avian life cycles and contained loss to farm produce. These viruses usually do not jump the species-animal barrier due to naturally-instituted susceptibility barriers with a restricted ability to multiply in men. Several factors may play a role. Vast genetic difference, for instance between birds and mammals tend to restrict reproducibility of the avian virus in a genetically diverse host. Avian influenza strains are internalized and transmitted via the α 2-3 receptors lining the respiratory tracts of vulnerable animals like ducks, geese, chicken and other birds; these receptors are not found in humans (who have the structurally different α 2-6 receptors instead) and thus should not be at risk from sick fowl.

The concern over the potency of the H5N1 strain of avian influenza arose a few years back with the turn of the century, with observations that avian viruses seemingly have attained the capability to circumvent some of these natural barriers. With repeated genetic reassortment under the pressure of natural selection, the avian influenza viral strains have progressively remodeled their structural proteins (HA and NA) which have evolved to become not too dissimilar to their human counterparts recognized previously to have caused pandemics, thus lowering the threshold for jumping the species barrier and afflicting humans. Such modified strains would have high "fatality-kill" rates during an infection as the human immune system would not been unexposed to such "novel" virus strains and unaccustomed to mount an adequate immune response to the invasion of these microbes, rendering the human host highly vulnerable (Figure 2). Other potential circumstances in which the avian influenza virus may potentially attain a more "humanized" predisposition have also been examined and reported (Figure 3). The pig/swine is a potential intermediary "mixing vessel" — this

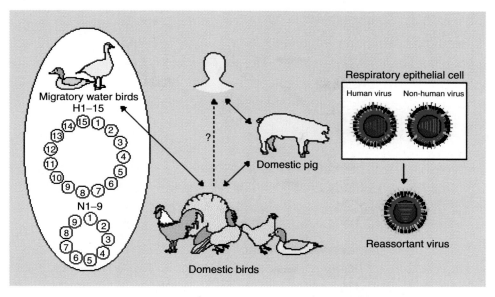

Figure 2: Origin of antigenic shift and pandemic influenza. The segmented nature of the influenza A genome, which has eight genes, facilitates reassortment; up to 256 gene combinations are possible during coinfection with human and non-human viruses. Antigenic shift can arise when genes encoding at least the hemagglutinin surface glycoprotein are introduced into people, by direct transmission of an avian virus from birds, as occurred with H5N1 virus, or after genetic reassortment is pigs, which support the growth of both avian and human viruses. Reprinted from *The Lancet*, Vol. 362, Nicholson, Wood, and Zambon: "Influenza," pp. 1733–1745, © 2003, with permission from Elsevier.

mammal is known to possess both the α 2-3 and α 2-6 receptors, rendering it susceptible to both human and avian viruses. Itself is not an uncommon sight in the home backyard farms of many-an-Asian families bred together with other domesticated fowl animals like chicken, duck and geese. Being subject to close exposure to both man and birds alike, simultaneous infection by both human and avian influenza strains is not unlikely, providing opportunity for both viruses to recombine and reassort to potentially produce a novel avian influenza strain capable of infecting humans (scenario A). Even in the absence of a co-infection, the avian influenza strain may mutate in an appropriate "universal host" and acquire the ability to overcome the species-barrier (scenario B). A more frightening spectre, though, lies in the ability of the avian strain to become highly infectious without going through an intermediary host — the remote scenario (C) whereby a poorly adaptable avian influenza strain infects a single human host having a concurrent human

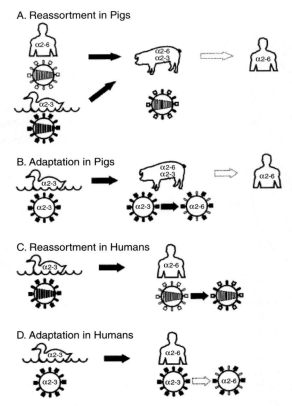

Figure 3: Models for the generation of pandemic influenza virus strains in pigs. Reprinted from *Clinical Microbiology Reviews*, Vol. 14, Horimoto and Kawaoka: "Pandemic threat posed by avian influenza A viruses," pp. 129–149, © 2001, with permission from the American Society for Microbiology.

influenza infection, reassorts within the latter and becomes highly infectious to men by acquiring the ability to transmit via the α 2-6 receptor path while retaining its potency. Such is the rationale for recommendations on influenza immunization — not as prevention for the avian strains, but for reducing opportunities for co-infections and subsequent mutations. Lastly, the prospect of a human host (scenario D), infected possibly by direct close proximity to an infected fowl, following which the avian strain (though initially less adaptable) undergoes mutation and re-adaptation to the human host environment to transmit with much greater ease and potency to other humans subsequently.

Alarmingly, recent analysis of the H1N1 strain of the Great Spanish Influenza Pandemic made possible by advances in molecular technology revealed that the 1917–18 strain was, in fact, a spontaneous mutation of a pure avian strain and not a result of reassortment. The implication of which is that history might again, at some point repeat itself.

Prior Outbreaks of Avian Influenza Until Recently

Avian influenza viruses of certain hemagglutinin subtypes — H5 and H7 have been known to cause human disease and limited outbreaks under the above circumstances. The telling event occurred in 1997 in Hong Kong in which an outbreak of H5N1 resulted in 18 human infections with a 50% mortality. The index patients were then, all exposed to live poultry. A smaller outbreak occurred in 2003, but this masked by the news-grabbing Severe Acute Respiratory Syndrome (SARS) outbreak which was happening simultaneously in Hong Kong. An outbreak of H7N7 was reported in Holland in 2003, afflicting more than 80 patients presenting mainly with conjunctivitis, but with one fatality. Isolated cases of H7N2 and H9N2 infection in New York and Hong Kong also followed, until the current H5N1 outbreak in Asia from 2004 … …

Transmissibility

Human influenza is transmitted by the inhalation of airborne secretions and infectious respiratory droplets (invisible to the naked eye) released by infected individuals as they breathe. It likely can also be acquired by direct contact with infected individuals or even with contaminated inanimate objects previously touched by sick individuals with direct inoculation into the patient's body. The challenge in limiting the transmissibility of influenza lies in that the virus is being shed by the afflicted even before the symptoms are experienced; *viz* the individual may be infectious even before he or she becomes febrile or has symptoms of cough and lethargy. This is further hampered by the finding that certain individuals especially children may continue to shed the virus for as long as 21 days, though for most adults, the virus is usually not detectable after a week.

From the data available to date on the H5N1 human influenza A cases, which is happening in tandem with the widespread H5N1 avian influenza outbreaks in fowl and lifestock in Asia, the method of transmission is indicative of bird-to-human, and possibly environment-to-human spread. Animal-to-human spread has been the most consistent reported modality since 1997. Almost all human cases have ascertained exposure to direct close contact with infected poultry, ranging with handling and playing with infected birds, feather-plucking and preparation of poultry for consumption, eating of raw or poorly cooked animal parts. Transmission has been attributed to close droplet inhalation and direct inoculation under such conditions. Possible human-to-human transmission has been raised in a handful of cases whereby close intimate contact with household members providing care for sick family members was the only exposure contact history identified. Healthcare workers attending to such infected patients have to date, not succumbed to the disease, even in the absence of protective gear, though there had been some suggestive indication that their immune system had been challenged by the H5N1 virus as indicated by blood testing. Visitors to outbreak regions have not been reportedly infected. However, recent cases, especially in China, whereby definite epidemiological exposure to either infected animals or individuals could not be ascertained at all in a few cases of apparent H5N1 infection, has raised concern further unestablished methods of spread.

Limited transmission capability, as it may appear though, for the H5N1 avian influenza virus in humans at this point in time; the fundamental concern, as discussed in the preceding section, lies in the unpredictable instant when the avian H5N1 virus in an infected human, by chance of natural mutation, acquires the adaptability of human influenza strains to transmit with ease within the population while retaining most of its genetic uniqueness to pose a new challenge to the unprimed human immune system, sparking the initial flame to an unquenchable fire of influenza pandemic worldwide.

Illness Symptomatology

Like the Great Pandemic of 1917–18, most cases of human H5N1 infections involved previously healthy young individuals. The following data are collected from H5N1 patient cohorts in Hong Kong, Thailand, Vietnam and Cambodia as published recently in the September 2005 issue of the *New England Journal of Medicine* (Table 1). The time to onset of illness after presumptive exposure had ranged from two days to an excess of eight days. Almost all patients present initially with fever of more than 38°C with cough and subsequently shortness of breath, with occasional headaches and muscular aches. Running nose and sore throat, as would be anticipated in a non-influenza upper respiratory tract infection, are not prominent features. Sputum production is variable. Diarrhoea, vomiting and abdominal pain have also been reported. Most patients present to the hospital almost up

Table 1: Presentation and outcomes among patients with confirmed avian influenza A (H5N1).*

Outcome of Measure	Hong Kong, 1997 (N = 18)	Thailand, 2004 (N = 17)	Vietnam, 2004 (N = 10)	Ho Chi Minh City, 2005 (N = 10)	Cambodia, 2005 (N = 4)
Age — yr					
Median	9.5	14	13.7[†]	19.4[†]	22
Range	1–60	2–58	5–24	6–35	8–28
Male sex — no. (%)	8 (44)	9 (53)	6 (60)	3 (30)	1 (25)
Time from last presumed exposure to onset of illness — days					
Median	NS	4	3	NS	NS
Range		2–8	2–4		
No. of family clusters		1	2	1	1
Patients with exposure to ill poultry — no./total no. (%)	11/16 (70) visited poultry markets	14/17 (82)	8/9 (89)	6/6 (100) Status of 4 unknown	3/4 (75)
Time from onset of illness to presentation or hospitalization — days					
Median	3	NS	6	6	8[‡]
Range	1–7		3–8	4–7	5–8
Clinical presentation — no./total no. (%)					
Fever (temperature > 38°C)	17/18 (94)	17/17(100)	10/10 (100)	10/10 (100)	4/4 (100)
Headache	4/18 (22)	NS	NS	1/10 (10)	4/14 (100)
Myalgia	2/18 (11)	9/17 (53)	0	2/10 (20)	NS
Diarrhea	3/18 (17)	7/17 (41)	7/10 (70)	NS	2/4 (50)
Abdominal pain	3/18 (17)	4/17 (24)	NS	NS	2/4 (50)
Vomiting	6/18 (33)	4/17 (24)	NS	1/10 (10)	0
Cough[§]	12/18 (67)	16/17 (94)	10/10 (100)	10/10 (100)	4/4 (100)
Sputum	NS	13/17 (76)	5/10 (50)	3/10 (30)	NS
Sore throat	4/12 (33)	12/17 (72)	0	0	1/4 (25)
Rhinorrhea	7/12 (58)	9/17 (53)	0	0	NS
Shortness of breath[§]	1/18 (6)	13/17 (76)	10/10 (100)	10/10 (100)	NS
Pulmonary infiltrates	11/18 (61)	17/17 (100)	10/10 (100)	10/10 (100)	4/4 (100)
Lymphopenia[¶]	11/18 (61)	7/17 (58)	NS	8/10 (80)	1/2 (50)
Thrombocytopenia	NS	4/12 (33)	NS	8/10 (80)	1/2 (50)
Increased aminotransferase levels	11/18 (61)	8/12 (67)	5/6 (83)	7/10 (70)	NS
Hospital course — no. (%)					
Respiratory failure	8 (44)	13 (76)	9 (90)	7 (70)	4 (100)
Cardiac failure	NS	7 (41)	NS	0	NS
Renal dysfunction	4 (22)	5 (29)	1 (10)	2 (20)	NS
Antiviral therapy[‖]					
Amantadine	10 (56)	0	0	0	NS
Ribavirin	1 (6)	0	2 (20)	0	
Oseltamivir	0	10 (59)	5 (50)	10 (100)	

Table 1: (*Continued*)

Outcome of Measure	Hong Kong, 1997 (N = 18)	Thailand, 2004 (N = 17)	Vietnam, 2004 (N = 10)	Ho Chi Minh City, 2005 (N = 10)	Cambodia, 2005 (N = 4)
Corticosteroids**	5 (28)	8 (47)	7 (70)	5 (50)	NS
Inotropoc agents	NS	8 (47)	2 (20)	NS	
Time from onset of illness to death — days					
Median	23	12	9	12.8[†]	8
Range	8–29	9–30	4–17	4–21	6–10
Deaths — no. (%)	6 (33)	12 (71)	8 (80)	8 (80)	4 (100)

*Data from Hong Kong are from Yuen *et al.*,[1] and Chan,[2] data on Thailand are from Chotpitaya-sunondh *et al.*,[3] data on Vietnam are from Hien *et al.*,[4] or data were presented at the WHO Consultation. NS denotes not stated.

[†]The median was unavailable, and the mean is given.

[‡]Some patients had multiple outpatient illness visits before hospitalization.

[§]In Hong Kong, shortness of breath later developed in 11 of 18 patients (61 percent) during hospitalization. In Thailand, all patients had cough and shortness of breath at hospitalization.

[¶]In Vietnam, the median lymphocyte count was 700 per cubic millimeter (range, 250 to 1100), and the median leukocyte count was 2100 per cubic millimeter (range, 1200 to 3400).[4] In Thailand, the mean leukocyte count was 4900 per cubic millimeter (range, 1200 to 13,600),[3] and the lymphocyte count was 1453 per cubic millimeter (range, 454 to 3400).

[||]In Thailand, 7 of 10 patients given oseltamivir died a mean of 11 days after the onset of symptoms (range, 5 to 22 days), as compared with 5 of 7 untreated patients. Oseltamivir was used in conventional doses (75 mg orally, twice daily for 5 to 10 days with a weight-based dose reduction in children) in the majority of recipients. In Vietnam, one of five recipients of oseltamivir recovered, as compared with one of five untreated patients.[4] The use of relatively low doses of oral ribavirin in two patients was not associated with obvious effectiveness.

**Initial patients in Vietnam received methylprednisolone (5 mg per kilogram of body weight per day or 1 to 2 mg per kilogram) for one to four days;[4] subsequent patients in Ho Chi Minh City received dexamethasone at 0.4 mg per kilogram per day for five days in a randomized trial. In Thailand, methylprednisolone (2 mg per kilogram per day) was administered for two to five days.

Source: *New England Journal of Medicine* 2005;353(13):1374–1385 (29 September 2005). Copyright © 2006 Massachusetts Medical Society. All rights reserved.

to about a week after onset of symptoms, upon which most would have developed non-specific changes on chest X-ray which could have been no little difference in appearance even to the expert eye from a routine bacterial pneumonia.

The crux of the difficult challenge in diagnosing H5N1 infection lies in its non-specific presentation. As can be alluded above, the symptomatology is non-specific, and is shared by the more commonly encountered upper respiratory tract infection and bacterial pneumonia in medical practice. Chest X-ray findings are not specific. Basic laboratory tests may merely indicate a mildly depressed white cell and platelet count. Ascertaining epidemiological exposure is time-consuming and may not be apparent at initial physician-patient contact. In a non-pandemic setting, a high level of suspicion may be the only reliable guard for cost-effective investigation of suspect cases, as specific diagnosis of confirmed H5N1 infection requires specialized molecular tests (polymerase chain reactions/PCRs) which may not be readily available in the vast lands of such developing countries whereby H5N1 avian infection is currently endemic.

With progressive disease, patients who are unable to mount an adequate immune response to the viral invasion will go into multiorgan failure requiring assisted ventilation and admission to an intensive care unit. Supportive therapy with broad spectrum antibiotics, antiviral agents have been administered with variable success. Reported overall mortally rates can stand at in excess of 80%.

Antiviral Agents

Logically, mode of action of antiviral drugs would be targeted at sites responsible for virus growth and duplication. For human influenza infection, two classes of drugs are currently available: the amantanes (amantadine and rimantadine) and the newer class of neuraminidase (NA) inhibitors (zanamivir [Relenza®] and oseltamivir [Tamiflu®]). The amantanes interfere with viral uncoating within the cell but are ineffective against the current avian H5N1 viruses. Thus, the neuraminidase inhibitors remain possibly the main treatment and possibly the prevention option against avian influenza. These drugs inactivate the NA protein on the surface of the influenza virus, restricting its ability to release "baby viruses" or virions to infect other human cells, clipping its reproductive potential and halting its spread (Figure 4). Zanamivir is administered by oral inhalation directly into the respiratory tract while oseltamivir is more conveniently taken orally.

It is pertinent to point out that in the drug trials involving neuraminidase inhibitors in human influenza, zanamivir or oseltamivir administered within 48 hours of illness onset served only to decrease length of illness by one to two days. The implication is that they are not the "magic bullet" nor the panacea, especially to the H5N1 human influenza as the drugs do not instantaneously eradicate viremia. The disease will continue to run its course, albeit at hopefully, a less intense severity. Recent reports of H5N1 virus strains with mutations conferring high level resistance to oseltamivir in two Vietnamese patients who eventually succumbed to the disease have further raised concern on the adequacy of our armamentarium. This is not an unexpected development, as it has been noted that influenza A (H1N1 and H3N2) strains have been known to develop drug resistant variants in patients who receive oseltamivir, especially children.

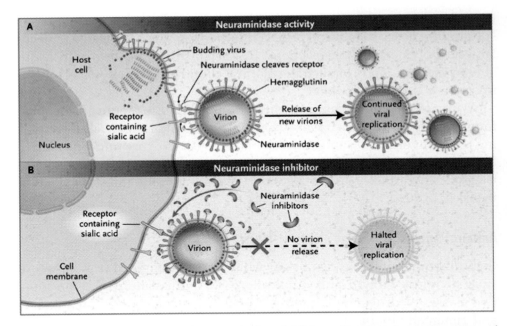

Figure 4: Mechanism of action of neuraminidase inhibitors. Panel A shows the action of neuraminidase in the continued replicaiton of virions in influenza infection. The replication is blocked by neuraminidase inhibitors (Panel B), which prevent virions from being released from the surface of infected cells. *Source: New England Journal of Medicine*, 2005; 353(13):1363–1373 (29 September 2005). Copyright © 2006 Massachusetts Medical Society. All rights reserved.

Nonetheless, neuraminidase inhibitors do have its place and forms part of the strategy in dealing with an avian influenza pandemic. Controversy remains as to whether oseltamivir or even zanamivir should be prescribed by the physician on demand for (avian) influenza prophylaxis. The current supply of oseltamivir is likely to be inadequate in the event of an avian influenza pandemic. It is the opinion of most experts that personal stockpiling of oseltamivir under such circumstances depletes supply to patients who would really benefit from the drug, and unnecessary use (without directions from the relevant medical experts) creates opportunities for development of drug resistance. For some, they may have only one chance with oseltamivir, so usage has to be prudent.

Vaccine Development

There are currently no commercially available vaccines for prevention specifically against human H5N1 infections. However, the grim prospects of a looming pandemic have propelled research bodies and pharmaceutical industries in developing potential vaccines via cutting edge genetical techniques. These candidate vaccines are currently undergoing preliminary trials and if proven to be eventually effective, will be launched into large scale production. However, should the outbreak occur in the months ahead, even if the pharmaceutical industry launches full time into production of a viable vaccine, there would likely be an insufficient supply for the countries most in need.

Recommendations remain though, by the World Health Organization (WHO) for susceptible individuals to continue receiving their annual influenza vaccination against endemic circulating influenza A H1N1 and H3N2 strains, as well as influenza B virus in the form of a 3-in-1 injectable preparation. Disease burden with non-H5 influenza A-attributable illness worldwide remains significant and overwhelming as compared to the current number of H5N1 human cases scattered in Asia. Immunization is also thought to minimize the potential risk of a co-infection with a H5N1 strain in permitting the remote opportunity of adaptation of the latter within the human host.

Conclusion

The spectre of an influenza pandemic continues to loom in the foreground. As with lessons learnt with other infectious disease outbreaks that have come and gone, understanding of the potential enemy and preparedness remain our best guard against a repeat of history.

References

1. Yuen KY, Chan PK, Peiris M, *et al.* Clinical features and rapid viral diagnosis of human disease associated with avian influenza A H5N1 virus. *Lancet* 1998;351:467–471.
2. Chan PK. Outbreak of avian influenza A(H5N1) virus infection in Hong Kong in 1997. *Clin Infect Dis* 2002;34(Suppl 2):S58–S64.
3. Chotpitayasunondh T, Ungchusak K, Hanshaoworakul W, *et al.* Human disease from influenza A (H5N1), Thailand, 2004. *Emerg Infect Dis* 2005;11:201–209.
4. Hien TT, Liem NT, Dung NT, *et al.* Avian influenza A (H5N1) in 10 patients in Vietnam. *N Engl J Med* 2004;350:1179–1188.

2

Virology View

Paul K.-S. Chan

The influenza virus is structurally a changing creature and ecologically a master of metamorphosis. As an individual virus particle, it utilizes an unfaithful replication enzyme which is bound to produce mutations in its progeny. When such mutations have accumulated to an extent large enough to fool the human immune system, we will experience a heavy wave of flu season. This occurs once every few years. It is now well-documented that these flu waves are associated with excess mortality. However, what is of more serious concern is the unique behavior of the virus population as a whole. Influenza virus infects not only humans, but other mammals and more importantly the bird species. There is a species barrier where virus subtypes circulating within one species cannot cross-infect other species. For instance, human infections are largely confined to two subtypes, H1N1 and H3N2, and our immune system is naïve to other subtypes that are circulating for example within the bird species. The ecology of influenza virus is not to the favor of human beings. While humans have only experienced a restricted number of influenza sub-types, all subtypes are found circulating in the waterfowls (16 different hemagglutinins and nine different neuraminidases) in nature. With this ecology, human beings are at a continuous threat of being bombarded by novel influenza subtypes introduced from the bird species. Once a

(Continued)

15

(Continued)

particular superstrain of the virus overcomes the species barrier, the whole world will have to face an infection that can easily be transmitted by sneezing and coughing, and to which our immune system has never experienced before. This exceptional victory of influenza virus has happened in three painful occasions within the last century causing more damages than a world war. Many virologists believe that the next disaster, an influenza pandemic, is imminent.

What Does H5N1 Stand For?

The outermost layer of an influenza virus particle, referred to as the "envelope," comprises of three proteins. Two of them, the hemagglutinin (H) and neuraminidase (N) proteins, are used for classifying and naming the virus, e.g. H5N1, H3N2 and H1N1. Hemagglutinin serves as the first contact point between the virus and the target host cell. It plays the role of a key in opening the door for entering into the host cell. This door opening process, referred as "receptor-binding," is a very specific process, i.e. the virus has to acquire the right hemagglutinin before it can establish an infection in the cells of a certain animal species. This key-lock matching is one of the critical barriers preventing transmission of avian influenza subtypes, e.g. H5, to humans. The neuraminidase serves as a pair of scissors to cleave viruses from mucus secretion in the respiratory tract so that the viruses can move freely to find other cells to establish a new round of infection. This cleavage function of the neuraminidase is also important for releasing mature virus particles from the infected host cell surface.

At present, 16 different kinds of hemagglutinin and nine different kinds of neuraminidase are known to exist. Each influenza virus only harbors one kind of hemagglutinin and one kind of neuraminidase. For instance, the influenza viruses circulating in humans that cause seasonal flu are H3N2 and H1N1. Viruses that are normally restricted to bird species but have occasionally crossed the species barrier to infect humans include H9N2, H7N7 and H7N3. H5N1 is by far the most alarming avian influenza subtype which has caused widespread poultry outbreaks since late 2003 (Figure 1).

What Makes the Influenza Virus So Special?

While viruses are the smallest microorganisms known to date, they are certainly not the simplest. The structure, characteristics, biology and

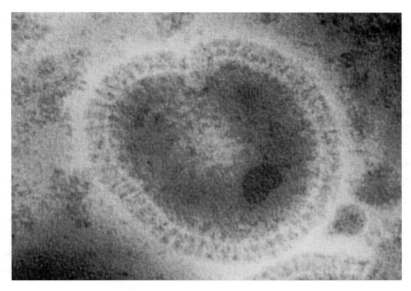

Figure 1: An electron micrograph of influenza virus. The appearance of influenza virus particles of different subtypes, e.g. H3N2, H1N1 and H5N1 are indistinguishable from each other. They are very tiny particles of sizes ranging from 80–120 nm in diameter. The fringe seen in the diagram comprise of two important proteins, the hemagglutinin (H) and the neuraminidase (N), which are critical in determining the characteristics of the virus, and are used for naming the virus.

physiology of an organism is governed by its genetic code carried in a double-stranded helix of deoxyribonucleic acid (DNA). It is most important for an organism to make an exact copy of this DNA for its daughter cells during the process of cell division, otherwise its characteristics may change in the new generation. Some viruses use DNA to carry their genetic codes, while others like the influenza virus utilize RNA to carry genetic codes. RNA is not the preferred means to carry genetic codes as it relies on a primitive enzyme, RNA polymerase, to reproduce itself. This RNA polymerase in contrast to those used for replicating DNA molecules, does not have a proof reading capacity. In other words, RNA viruses like influenza have a much higher chance of producing a slightly different offspring due to the increased error rate associated with the replicating enzyme being used. The chance of error has been estimated to be around one per ten thousand of bases. When these slight changes have accumulated to a certain degree and have occurred in critical positions, it may affect the outcome of an infection. For example, our immune system may not be able to "recognize" the virus, and thus will take a longer time to control the infection, as if it is being exposed to it for the first time. This phenomenon of continuous "change or mutation" which is an intrinsic property of influenza virus is technically referred as "antigenic drift." This explains why once in a few years, we experience a more severe attack of flu season.

While a bad flu season due to a substantial antigenic drift causes significant mortality and morbidity, this is not the most threatening issue concerning influenza. What is more worying is a scenario of the change in the property of the virus not acquired through a graduate process, i.e. point mutations, but rather arises so suddenly that the human immune system is completely naïve to. The way that influenza virus carries its genetic code also paths such possibility. A vast majority of viruses carry their genetic code in a continuous fragment of DNA or RNA. However, the genetic code of influenza viruses is encrypted in eight separate fragments. Imagine when influenza viruses from different sources, e.g. human and bird, establish an infection simultaneously in the same host, e.g. pig; these two viruses can exchange their genetic segments. The progeny viruses can have combinations of gene segments ranging from zero to eight segments originating from the bird virus, and vice versa from the human virus. With this, the change in genetic make-up is not just a few points but the whole trunk of the genetic code. This swapping of genetic segments is referred to as "reassortment," which results in a sudden and drastic change in the property of the virus known. This phenomenon is technically known as "antigenic shift" (Figure 2).

Why Birds are Important?

A few other virus families also employ a segmented genome, but they do not have the potential to cause a pandemic (defined as an infection spreading to multiple regions within a short period of time). It is the peculiar ecology of influenza, in addition to its segmented genome, that confers its potential for causing a pandemic. Imagine when two almost identical viruses exchange their genetic segments, the progeny viruses will still be very similar to their parents. However, if the parents are quite different, the offspring that has acquired a few genetic segments from one parent, and a few from the other would then have characteristics of a very large difference from either parent. The scenario of influenza ecology is that there are a limited number of virus subtypes, currently H3N2 and H1N1, circulating within the human population. These viruses are highly adapted to humans, and in particular, these viruses can be transmitted very efficiently between humans. Influenza viruses also circulate in many other animal species including horses, pigs, sea mammals and birds. Wild waterfowls are the principal

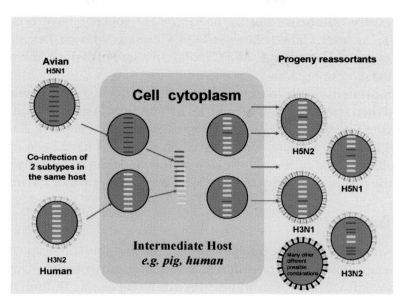

Figure 2: Reassortment of influenza viruses. Each influenza virus particle contains eight segments of genetic materials. The constituent of these genetic segments determine the property of the virus. Genetic segments of avian viruses are very different from those found in human viruses. If both human and avian influenza viruses have a chance to establish an infection in the same host, exchange of these genetic segments becomes possible. Many different combinations of mixing of genetic segments can be found in the progeny viruses. Some of these may not survive whereas others can further propagate in a new host. If one of these reassortants can be transmitted efficiently from human to human, an influenza pandemic may occur.

natural reservoir for influenza viruses. Waterfowls do not suffer from the infection, and yet a large amount of viruses are shed from their droppings. Furthermore, all the known 16 types of hemagglutinin (H) and nine types of neuraminidase (N) can be found from avian influenza viruses circulating among waterfowls. Therefore, waterfowls are the natural playground for influenza viruses allowing mixing and exchanging of gene segments. The H5N1 virus causing a few large poultry outbreaks and 18 human infections with six deaths in Hong Kong in 1997 was a reassortant from a goose virus (H5N1), a quail virus (H9N2), and a teal virus (H6N1).

Water birds serve as a gene pool for generating new viruses, but they seldom suffer from the infection. When these viruses are transmitted to land birds, they sometimes suffer from the infection. The "fowl plaque" was first described in 1878 as a disease affecting chickens in Italy. The condition is now known to be caused by highly pathogenic avian influenza viruses. Fowl plaque is still a major concern for the poultry industry. Over the last 30 years, many poultry outbreaks due to the H5 or H7 subtype have occurred in Australia, England, United States, Ireland, Germany, Mexico, Pakistan, Italy, Hong Kong, the Netherlands and Canada. In a few occasions, the infection has spilled over to humans.

The most remarkable recent poultry outbreak due to H5N1 started in late 2003 and then spread to many countries in Southeast Asia in 2004, and have extended to Europe in 2005, and Africa in 2006. Up to February 2006, more than 160 human infections with more than 80 deaths have been recorded. This multi-regional outbreak of avian influenza virus has clearly demonstrated the role of migratory birds in long-distance spread of the infection.

What is the Role of Pigs?

Waterfowls serve as a gene pool housing all the possible subtypes (16 different hemagglutinins and nine different neuraminidases) of influenza viruses. Only a few influenza virus subtypes (three different hemagglutinins and two different neuraminidases) have been successfully circulated in humans. It is known that avian influenza viruses replicate poorly in humans, and human viruses replicate poorly in birds. In such instances, how does the avian virus find a chance to exchange its genetic segments (reassortment) with those of human influenza viruses? This reassortment between avian and human influenza can only happen when there is a host that can be infected by both influenza subtypes, i.e. a mixing vessel. Pigs seem to be at least one of the animal species that are readily infected by human and avian influenza viruses. Pigs contain cellular receptors utilized by human influenza viruses as well as those utilized by avian viruses. There is also scientific evidence to suggest that repeated replication of avian viruses in pigs may lead to changes resulting in a more human-like virus. The concept that an intermediate host, like pig, is essential for generating a novel influenza strain with a high human-to-human transmission efficiency, thus a pandemic capacity, is well accepted. In fact, it accounts for the two most recent influenza pandemics that happened in 1957 and 1968. The 1918 pandemic has been assumed to be the result of reassortment between human and avian viruses. However, recent studies have provided convincing evidence to support that the 1918 pandemic virus was in fact a direct adaptation to human transmission as result of mutations over critical positions of an avian virus, rather than reassortment. With these information, it is now clear that avian influenza viruses can breach the species barrier either by reassortment with an existing human virus or by acquiring certain critical mutations that allow adaptation for replication and transmission in humans (Figure 2).

Is it Only H5N1 or Something Else?

Human infection with avian influenza virus H5N1 was first recognized in Hong Kong in 1997 following multiple poultry outbreaks. It was due to direct transmission from poultry to humans without prior reassortment in an intermediate host. After this initial attack which caused six deaths, the virus re-emerged again in 2003 infecting a family in Hong Kong. Whether the source of this outbreak originated in Fujian (mainland China) or Hong Kong is still a mystery.

In mid-December 2003, a large poultry outbreak of H5N1 affecting more than 19,000 chickens occurred in Eumsung district, near the capital city of Seoul. The outbreak evolved quickly over the next two weeks spreading to other chicken and duck farms in five provinces in the Republic of Korea, where at least 1.5 million birds have died. Poultry outbreaks of H5N1 were subsequently observed in multiple countries including Cambodia, China, Indonesia, Japan, Laos, South Korea, Thailand and Vietnam, killing hundreds of millions of birds in the region. As with the incidence of the H5N1 outbreak in Hong Kong in 1997, this regional wide poultry outbreak of H5N1 also associated with occasional transmission to humans. As at February 2006, more than 160 human infections with more than 80 deaths due to avian influenza virus H5N1 have been recorded. With this history, H5N1 is certainly an avian virus with a high potential to emerge as the next pandemic virus. Nevertheless, H5N1 is not the only avian virus with such potential.

What About H9N2?

Avian influenza virus H9N2 has also occasionally succeeded in establishing infections in humans. Two young children infected with H9N2 were detected in Hong Kong in 1999, and another child in 2003. All three children recovered after a mild course of upper respiratory tract illness. Subsequent surveillance indicated a minute proportion of Hong Kong people have been exposed to the virus, most probably with asymptomatic or with mild symptoms. While currently there is no evidence of efficient human-to-human transmission of H9N2, its potential of emerging to such a stage should not be neglected. As infected birds and infected humans only suffer from mild symptoms or even without any signs of illness, this makes it even more difficult to trace the path of this virus. Therefore, H9N2 may enjoy a bigger window in its adaptation to human infection and transmission. One may argue that if the illnesses caused by H9N2 in birds and humans are so mild, why should we bother? There are at least two concerns that we should not ignore the importance of H9N2. Firstly, the previous mild human infections of H9N2 were due to a non-adapted virus for which the replication intensity that can be achieved in human is very low. Virus replication is most probably restricted to a small number of cells within the upper respiratory tract, and thus are only associated with mild symptoms. However, if the virus can, after adaptation, replicate more efficiently and extend further within or even outside the respiratory tract, the clinical consequences could be completely different. One should not forget that the human immune system is naïve to this virus. The second scenario is that H9N2 may remain mild even after adaptation in humans, which means this H9N2 virus carrying the characteristics of avian viruses will be circulating and continuously infecting a substantial proportion of people. H9N2 would then have many chances to exchange its genetic segments with the usual human influenza viruses H3N2 and H1N1. No one can guarantee this reassortment will not create a novel influenza strain with a high virulence as well as a high human-to-human transmission efficiency.

What Have the H7 Avian Viruses Done to Humans?

Avian influenza viruses can generally be classified into two groups according to their virulence in poultry. The more lethal ones are referred to as "highly pathogenic avian influenza (HPAI)," whereas those causing mild or no symptoms in poultry are referred to as "low pathogenicity avian influenza (LPAI)." The H5 and H7 subtypes are typical examples of highly pathogenic avian influenza viruses. The "fowl plaque" was first described in 1878 in Italy affecting chickens. Similar outbreaks were then observed in other parts of Europe and worldwide. In 1902, a virus, believed to be the causative agent, was isolated from a chicken. This first ever isolated influenza virus was later identified to be H7N7. H7N7 has been known for a long time that it can occasionally succeed in transmitting from birds to humans and in most situations the infections are presented as conjunctivitis. In one of the recent cases (detected in 1996 in England), the virus was isolated from a woman with conjunctivitis. The source of infection was considered to be waterfowls in a small lake. The most notable incidence occurred in 2003. An outbreak of H7N7 first started in the Netherlands which then spread to Germany and Belgium. Altogether 89 human infections were confirmed. The majority of the infected persons had conjunctivitis only, and a small proportion had mild influenza-like illnesses. However, a veterinarian died of acute respiratory distress syndrome. The virus isolated from this fatal case had some genetic differences compared to other mild cases, which may account for the unusual severity.

Another H7 subtype, H7N3, has also crossed the species barrier. This influenza subtype caused a large wave of poultry outbreaks in British Columbia, Canada. A widespread surveillance identified two human infections. Both of them recovered after a course of conjunctivitis and mild influenza-like illnesses.

The H7 avian influenza viruses are certainly potential candidates of the next pandemic virus.

What Viruses Have Caused Pandemics?

History tells facts. Over the last century, three pandemic influenza viruses have successfully emerged — the 1918 (Spanish influenza) H1N1 virus, the 1957 (Asian influenza) H2N2 virus, and the 1968 (Hong Kong influenza) H3N2 virus. While in each incidence, the human population was challenged by a novel infection, the overall impact varies quite a lot. Among the many different factors governing the outcome of a pandemic, e.g. human density and movement, availability of healthcare facilities, etc.; the virulence of the virus is a critical determinant.

It has been estimated that 20–50 million people died from the 1918 Spanish influenza virus. This astonishing death toll was much higher than the two subsequent pandemics. The nature of the 1918 virus and the reasons for such a high death rate have been a mystery for many years. It was not until 1933 that the influenza virus was first successfully isolated from humans. Therefore, virological information on human influenza circulating before 1933 was not easily obtained, if not impossible. However, with the recent advancement in molecular biology techniques, the whole 1918 virus was re-created in 2005 to unravel what happened a century ago. It has all along been assumed by most people that the 1918 virus was a reassortant from avian and human influenza viruses aroused in an intermediate host, most probably pig. However, after detailed analysis on the genetic sequences of the 1918 virus, it does not come to such a conclusion. Rather, the sequence data suggests that all the eight segments of the viral genome have originated from an avian influenza virus.

The purely avian origin of the 1918 virus provides an important explanation to the particularly high virulence of this virus compared to the 1957 and 1968 viruses. The H2N2 virus causing the pandemic in 1957 was a reassortant created from a human virus and an avian virus, as a result of the two viruses simultaneously infecting an intermediate host. This H2N2 has five gene segments derived from the human virus (i.e. the H1N1 circulating at that time) and three gene segments from the avian virus. Similarly, the H3N2 virus which caused the 1968 pandemic was also a reassortant created from a human and an avian virus. It contains two genetic segments from an avian source, six segments from the circulating human virus H2N2, of which five segments were carried over from the 1918 virus.

Conclusions

A century of history is still too short to draw any concrete predictions on influenza pandemics, as there have been, fortunately, only three episodes of such disaster. Nevertheless, a few observations are worth noting. The ability of influenza viruses to cause large pandemics resulting in severe human health and economic loss is given by nature. The virus itself has an intrinsic propensity to generate mutations and therefore changing its characteristics are necessary for exploring and adapting to new environments and hosts. Furthermore, the ecology given to this virus allows the existence of silent reservoirs, notable the waterfowls, to serve as a gene pool for manufacturing new forms of the virus. One has to realize that practically nothing can be done to change these laws of nature. It is conceivable that it is just a matter of time for a new form of influenza virus with pandemic capacity to emerge.

What should we learn from history? History tells us that there are two ways that influenza viruses can establish pandemics.

The first way is by reassortment in an intermediate host as in 1957 and 1968. We should therefore minimise, if not eliminate, the intermediate host, notably pigs, from contacting human and avian influenza viruses. Biosecurity and species segregation for pig farms should be pursued.

The second way is by direct adaptation to human replication and transmission. This would most probably require repeated contacts between the avian viruses with humans. One obvious and urgent action is the need to establish a good surveillance system for detecting poultry outbreaks, and have them curtailed promptly to eliminate human exposure to infected birds. The importance of live poultry markets as a mediator for incubating and transmitting the virus to humans should not be ignored.

The battle on influenza is not going to be a short one.
A continuous concerted effort is needed.

3

The First Cases of H5N1 Infection in the World

Rita Y.-T. Sung

The Mysterious New Virus H5N1 Killed our Young Patient

I can never forget the year of 1997 — other than the historical event of the return of Hong Kong to China by the British Government, there was the other more personal reason of the unexpected death of one of our patients from a new emerging disease. The mysterious nature of the disease still haunts me from time to time. I remember vividly that the patient died a few days before Christmas, her prolonged coma in the Intensive Care Unit and final inevitable death made us very sad in the usually joyous holiday season. The patient was a 13-year-old, previously healthy girl. She began with flu-like symptoms: fever, sore throat, runny nose and dry cough on 20 November 1997. She attended the Accident and Emergency Department on the fourth day of illness because of persistent fever. A diagnosis of upper respiratory tract infection was made in the A&E Department and then was discharged on panadol medication. However, the swinging high fever persisted, she was therefore brought to see a general practitioner on the same day and was given an injection of Rocephin and oral Globocef (both Rocephin and Globocef are third generation cephalosporins — powerful broad spectrum antibiotics). She showed no signs of improvement, so she attended A&E again on 26 November 1997 when a chest X-ray was taken, showing lobar pneumonia involving her right lower lung field. She was then admitted to the pediatric ward for further management.

On admission, a detailed history was taken which revealed no recent travel history or contact with patients or poultry. She was alert. Her body temperature was 38.7°C. She had no respiratory distress, but decreased breath sounds and crepitations were detected on auscultation over her right lung base indicating pneumonia. The blood test showed that her white cell and platelet counts were slightly low at 4.7×10^9/L and 62×10^9/L, respectively. Since the blood picture suggested viral pneumonia or atypical pneumonia (pneumonia caused by certain atypical pathogens such as mycoplasma, Chlamydia and Legionella) and the apparent lack of response to broad spectrum antibiotics in her case, she was treated with Clarithromycin (an antibiotic effective against atypical bacterial infection). By the way, mycoplasma pneumonia is very common in children and it usually responds very well to Clrithromycin. Unfortunately, she had no response to this treatment. Her fever persisted and she coughed out a small amount of blood-stained sputum the next day. At that juncture, penicillin-resistant pneumococcal infection was considered to be a possible alternative diagnosis and another antibiotic, Cefotaxime, was added to cover this infection. (Pneumococcus is one of the most common bacteria which can cause septicemia, pneumonia, meningitis, etc. This bacterium used to be very sensitive to penicillin, but penicillin-resistant strains surged in the past decade due to indiscriminate use of antibiotics in many parts of the world.) The girl's condition deteriorated during the day with increasing respiratory rate and distress and had to be admitted to the ICU in the evening. She required to be put on a ventilator to assist her breathing so to maintain the oxygen level in her blood six hours after being admitted to ICU. She had rapid deterioration over the following three days with multiple organ dysfunctions. The status in body temperature (Figure 1), pulse (Figure 2), respiratory rate (Figure 3), red blood cell count (Table 1), white blood cell count (Table 2), renal and liver function (Table 3), and X-ray film (Figure 4) was deteriorated. By that time, the blood culture result (which was negative) became available, but Influenza A antigen was detected in her nasopharyngeal aspirate. Unexpectedly, the Government Virus Unit informed us on 6 December 1997 that H5N1 was confirmed. With no experience in treating such an infection caused by this new strain of virus, we tried two antiviral agents — Amantadine and Ribavirin — but the results were disappointing and the girl died of intractable multiple organ failure on 21 December 1997.

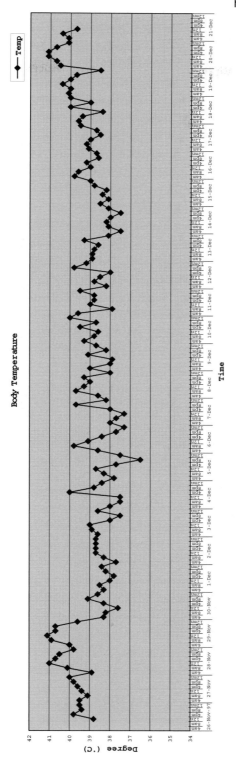

Figure 1: Body temperature chart.

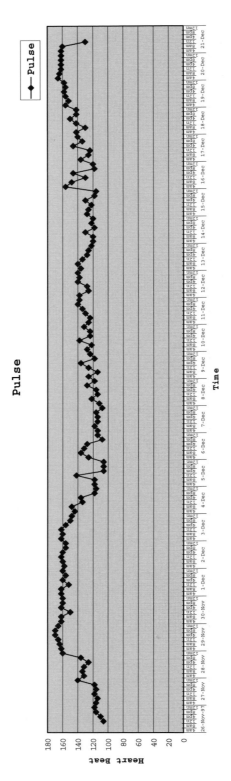

Figure 2: Pulse.

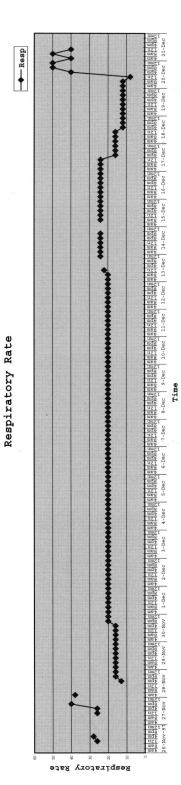

Figure 3: Respiratory rate.

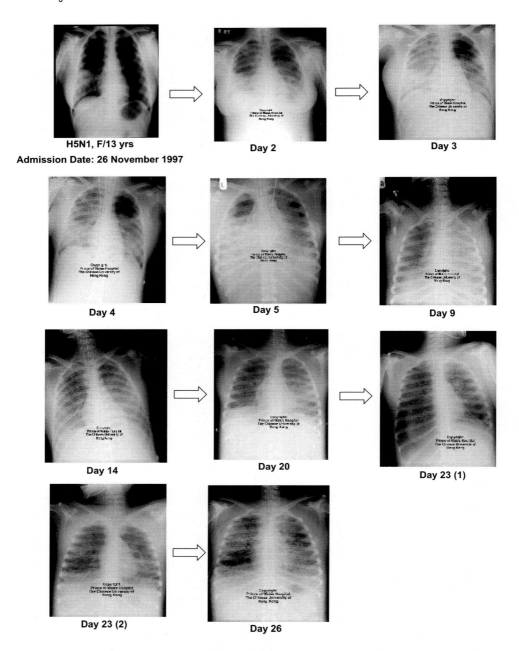

H5N1, F/13 yrs
Admission Date: 26 November 1997

Day 2

Day 3

Day 4

Day 5

Day 9

Day 14

Day 20

Day 23 (1)

Day 23 (2)

Day 26

Figure 4: X-ray film.

Table 1: Red blood cell count.

Date/ Reference range	Red cell count 3.70–4.90	Hemoglobin 11.5–4.3	HCT 0.32–0.43	MCV 81.0–97.0	MCH 27.0–32.0	MCHC 31.0–35.0
1997 Nov 27	4.65	14.2	0.431	92.6	30.4	32.8
Nov 28 (1)	3.93	11.8	0.361	91.9	30.0	32.7
Nov 28 (2)	3.81	11.4	0.352	92.5	29.9	32.3
Nov 29	2.95	8.8	0.269	91.1	29.8	32.7
Nov 29 (after blood transfusion)	4.31	13.0	0.394	91.2	30.0	32.9
Nov 30	4.33	13.1	0.384	88.8	30.4	34.2
Dec 1	3.34	10.3	0.301	90.2	30.9	34.2
Dec 2	2.83	8.7	0.253	89.4	30.8	34.4
Dec 3	2.10	6.5	0.187	89.1	30.9	34.6
Dec 4	2.12	6.7	0.192	90.8	31.5	34.7
Dec 5	2.80	8.4	0.247	88.1	30.1	34.2
Dec 6	2.62	7.9	0.232	88.6	30.2	34.1
Dec 7	2.90	8.2	0.242	83.4	28.2	33.8
Dec 8	2.69	7.4	0.229	85.2	27.3	32.1
Dec 9	2.66	7.6	0.233	87.4	28.7	32.8
Dec 10	2.76	7.8	0.245	88.8	28.3	31.8
Dec 11 (1)	2.78	8.0	0.243	87.4	28.8	32.9
Dec 11 (2)	2.54	7.1	0.216	84.8	33.0	28.0
Dec 12	3.05	8.2	0.256	83.8	26.9	32.1
Dec 13 (1)	2.98	8.7	0.245	82.5	29.1	35.3
Dec 13 (2)	3.26	9.5	0.275	84.3	29.1	34.5
Dec 13 (3)	3.17	9.3	0.270	85.0	29.3	34.4
Dec 14 (1)	3.6	10.8	0.307	85.3	29.9	35.1
Dec 14 (2)	3.16	9.5	0.274	86.6	30.0	34.6
Dec 15	3.54	10.5	0.313	88.3	29.7	33.6
Dec 16	3.36	10.1	0.292	87.0	29.9	34.4
Dec 17	2.23	6.4	0.196	87.6	28.8	32.9
Dec 18	3.70	10.9	0.321	86.7	29.5	34.0
Dec 19	3.48	10.3	0.306	87.9	29.6	33.6
Dec 20	2.91	8.7	0.252	86.6	30	34.7

This was the second fatal case of H5N1 in Hong Kong. The first was a three-year-old boy who died of multiple organ failure five days after admission into another hospital in May of the same year. H5N1 infection was only confirmed after his death. Since he was the first known case of a human contracting the H5N1 virus, the contribution of this infection to his death was not clear. Another confirmed H5N1 infection prior to our case occurred in November in a two-year old child with a small ventricular septal defect, he presented with mild upper respiratory tract infection and recovered without antiviral therapy. A full post-mortem examination revealed a deadly

Table 2: White blood cell count.

Date/ Reference range	Platelet count	White cell count	Neutrophils (%)	Lymphocytes (%)	Monocytes (%)	Eosinophils (%)	Basophils (%)
	140–380	4.0–10.8	41–73	19–47	4–10	1–6	0–1
1997 Nov 27	62	4.7	81	15	2	1	1
Nov 28 (1)	100	2.6	–	–	–	–	–
Nov 28 (2)	97	2.0	85	13	2	–	–
Nov 29	140	2.7	–	–	–	–	–
Nov 29 (after blood transfusion)	82	5.5	–	–	–	–	–
Nov 30	41	13.0	–	–	–	–	–
Dec 1	35	14.9	–	–	–	–	–
Dec 2	28	14.4	–	–	–	–	–
Dec 3	38	15.3	–	–	–	–	–
Dec 4	62	11.6	–	–	–	–	–
Dec 5	59	6.2	–	–	–	–	–
Dec 6	112	5.7	–	–	–	–	–
Dec 7	101	6.5	–	–	–	–	–
Dec 8	100	5.2	–	–	–	–	–
Dec 9	69	3.7	–	–	–	–	–
Dec 10	51	2.9	–	–	–	–	–
Dec 11 (1)	–	1.1	–	–	–	–	–
Dec 11 (2)	31	0.7	73	25	2	–	–
Dec 12	31	0.8	–	–	–	–	–
Dec 13 (1)	51	0.6	–	–	–	–	–
Dec 13 (2)	44	0.7	–	–	–	–	–
Dec 13 (3)	33	0.5	–	–	–	–	–
Dec 14 (1)	33	0.4	–	–	–	–	–
Dec 14 (2)	40	0.3	–	–	–	–	–
Dec 15	32	0.7	–	–	–	–	–
Dec 16	33	0.7	–	–	–	–	–
Dec 17	24	0.8	–	–	–	–	–
Dec 18	33	1.2	–	–	–	–	–
Dec 19	29	1.3	–	–	–	–	–
Dec 20	34	2.3	–	–	–	–	–

complication of H5N1 infection in our patient, namely Hemophagocytotic syndrome (the consumption of blood forming cells by the patients own white blood cells/macrophages/histiocytes). It was not until the death of our patient and concurrent admissions of similar cases to other hospitals that panic ensued amongst the health authorities and the public. The outbreak lasted for two months, a total of 17 cases were confirmed with five deaths. Their ages ranged from two to 60 years. Some of the patients had chronic illness while others were previously healthy. Half of the fatal cases were young and previously healthy. It ended in late December when the Hong Kong government made a decision to slaughter all the poultry in the farms and markets of Hong Kong. Eight years have passed since the first outbreak, the

Table 3: Renal and liver function.

Item \ Date	1997 Nov 28	1997 Dec 2	Reference range
Sodium	123	140	*134–145 mmol/l*
Potassium	3.6	4.4	*3.5–5.1 mmol/l*
Urea	2.0	20.1	*3.4–8.9 mmol/l*
Creatinine	56	367	*44–80 mmol/l*
Total protein	62	53	*66–81 g/l*
Albumin	27	22	*36–48 g/l*
Total bilirubin	7	10	*<15 umol/l*
Alk. phosphate	51	106	*105–335 U/l*
SGPT/ALT	38	40	*<58 U/l*
Calcium	1.95	1.93	*2.15–2.55 mmol/l*
Alb. adj. calcium	2.28	–	*2.15–2.55 mmol/l*
Phosphate	0.66	1.47	*0.82–1.4 mmol/l*

explanation for the dramatic difference in clinical outcomes, ranging from mild upper respiratory tract infection in some patients to severe pneumonia and multiple organ failure in others, remains a mystery.

4

The Second Phase After H5N1 Avian Influenza Virus Infection: The Three-Wave Spread in Thailand

Salin Chutinimitkul, Pattaratida Sa-nguanmoo and Yong Poovorawan

Influenza virus infection is a major public health problem around the globe. Worldwide, about 20% of children and 5% of adults develop symptomatic influenza A or B each year.[1] It is the cause of a broad range of illnesses, from less symptomatic infection to various respiratory syndromes and disorders effecting the lung, heart, brain, liver, kidneys and muscles. Most influenza infections are spread by virus burdened respiratory droplets that are expelled during coughing and sneezing. The initial site of replication is thought to be the tracheobronchial ciliated epithelium.[2] Influenza viruses are a member of the *Orthomyxoviridae* family, which are enveloped, single-stranded RNA viruses[3] and have segmented genomes that show great antigenic diversity. Influenza viruses are classified as types A, B and C based on differences in their nucleoproteins and matrix proteins. Of the three types of influenza viruses, only types A and B cause widespread outbreaks. Influenza A viruses are classified into subtypes based on antigenic differences between their two surface glycoproteins, hemagglutinin and neuraminidase. Serologically, 16 subtypes of HA (H1–H16) and nine subtypes of NA (N1–N9) have been identified.[4] All hemagglutinin and neuraminidase subtypes of viruses have been recovered from aquatic birds. In contrast, only three HA subtypes (H1, H2 and H3) and two NA subtypes (N1 and N2) have been commonly found in humans and routinely isolated since 1918.[5] Furthermore, the emergence of new influenza virus variants in the avian population has been reported to infect humans. In May and November–December 1997, 18 cases of influenza H5N1 infection were identified in people in Hong Kong.[6] The virus has since re-emerged in 2001–2002 and once more in February 2003, with two confirmed cases in a family of Hong Kong residents. After the H5N1 outbreak in Hong Kong, heightened surveillance in the adjoining Guangdong Province led to the recovery of nine human isolates of H9N2 virus during July–September 1998.[7] Avian H7N7 virus was first isolated in 1980 from four people who contracted purulent conjunctivitis when an infected animal sneezed into their faces.[8] An outbreak of highly pathogenic avian H7N7 influenza in poultry farms in the Netherlands, which began at the end of February 2003, was associated with fatal respiratory illness in one of 82 human cases by 21 April 2003.[9]

The Outbreak in Asia and the Three-Wave Outbreak in Thailand

H5N1 outbreak in Asia: An epidemic of avian influenza H5N1 strain has been reported in Asia since 1996, when the highly pathogenic H5N1 virus was isolated from a farmed goose in Guangdong Province, China. In 1997, human infections with H5N1 were reported in Hong Kong. Altogether, 18 cases (six fatal) were reported in the first known instance of human infection with this virus. Recently, H5N1 avian influenza has become epidemic in 13 countries in Asia, Republic of Korea, Vietnam, Japan, Cambodia, Lao PDR, Indonesia, China, Hong Kong, Malaysia, Iraq, Turkey, Mongolia and Thailand.[10] In addition, seven Asian countries, Vietnam, Indonesia, China, Cambodia, Iraq, Turkey and Thailand, identified H5N1 as the cause of human cases of severe respiratory disease with high fatality.[11] The genotype dominantly identified in poultry was genotype Z, which may offer the possibility of wild birds playing a role in the spread of this genotype, such that it has found a new ecological niche in poultry, but may not yet be fully adapted to this host.[12] Domestic ducks can act as silent reservoirs, excreting large quantities of highly pathogenic virus yet showing few if any signs of illness. Not only avian species have been reported, H5N1 infection in pigs was reported in China but there was no evidence to suggest that pig infections are widespread, and the finding appears to have limited epidemiological significance.[13] Apart from that, domestic cats experimentally infected with H5N1 develop severe disease and can spread infection to other cats.[14] In April 2005, wild birds begin dying at Qinghai Lake in central China, where hundreds of thousands of migratory birds congregate. Altogether, 6345 birds from different species died in the subsequent weeks. Viruses isolated from dead birds in Qinghai Lake suggests the outbreak, which was caused by a new H5N1 variant possibly carried along winter migratory routes, may be more lethal to wild birds and experimentally infected mice.[15]

Three-wave outbreak in Thailand: In Thailand, the avian influenza time-line can be split into three waves. In early January 2004 to mid-March 2004, nearly a hundred million domestic poultry have been slaughtered. Because of the distinctive feature of this virus which can cross from avian to human, 12 cases of human infection with eight fatalities have been seen. All 12 confirmed case-patients resided in villages that experienced abnormal chicken deaths, nine lived in households whose backyard chickens died, and eight reported direct contact with dead chickens. Seven were children less than 14 years of age. Fever preceded dyspnea by a median of five days, and lymphopenia significantly predicted acute respiratory distress syndrome development and death.[16] The second wave re-emerged in June/July 2004 to November 2004, in which five human cases occurred with four fatalities. A case report is published — indicating atypical human H5N1 infection in Thailand, with fever and diarrhea but no respiratory symptoms. The report suggests that the clinical spectrum of disease may be broader than previously thought.[17] Appallingly, an outbreak began in zoo tigers in Thailand said to have been fed chicken carcasses. Altogether, 147 tigers out of a population of 441 died or had to be euthanized. Avian influenza A (H5N1) virus caused severe pneumonia in tigers and leopards that fed on infected poultry carcasses[18] and this virus was attributed to a probable horizontal transmission among tigers.[19] This finding extends the host range of influenza virus and has implications for influenza virus epidemiology and wildlife conservation. In this second wave, the first published account of probable secondary human transmission of any avian influenza virus was reported. A young Thai girl with severe disease probably passed the virus to at least her mother, which resulted in a fatal disease.[20] In October 2005, the third wave outbreak was reported. As of early December 2005, five human cases, together with two fatalities were reported. The study that characterized the 2005 isolates recovered from chickens and quail in the same area of human cases showed the genetic drifts of the avian influenza isolates especially at the HA cleavage site, and H5N1 viruses have continued to evolve since early 2004 (unpublished data). The evolution of human and animal viruses circulating in Asia in 2005 suggests that several amino acids located near the receptor-binding site are undergoing change, some of which may affect antigenicity or transmissibility.[21]

Spread of the epidemic to Eurasia: The outbreak of avian influenza also spread to Eurasia since July 2005, with several new countries that had never reported epidemic of avian influenza previously. Russia, Kazakhstan, Mongolia, Romania, Ukraine, Croatia, Turkey and Iraq have now confirmed outbreaks of highly pathogenic avian influenza (HPAI), subsequently proved to be H5N1. There were 12 cases in Turkey with four deaths and one fatal case in Iraq.[22]

Genetic Evidence of Influenza A Virus Subtype H5N1

Influenza A viruses have been isolated from a diverse group of animals, including humans, pigs, horses, sea mammals and birds. All 16 HA and nine NA subtypes of type A viruses usually do not produce disease in wild aquatic bird populations, especially ducks, indicating influenza viruses are maintained with the optimal level of adaptation in this natural reservoir.[23] Recently, avian influenza virus subtypes H5N1, H7N7 and H9N2 have been reported to be directly transmitted to humans, raising the concern of a new influenza pandemic among the world's immunologically naive populations. Avian influenza viruses can be sorted on the basis of virulence: highly pathogenic avian influenza (HPAI) viruses cause systemic lethal infection, killing birds immediately 24 hours post-infection, and usually within one week, while low-pathogenic avian influenza (LPAI) viruses infrequently generate outbreaks of severe disease but with lower morbidity and mortality rates compared to those of HPAI viruses.[23] In January 2004, HPAI virus of the H5N1 subtype was first confirmed in poultry and humans in Thailand. Poultry populations in 1417 villages in 60 of 76 provinces were affected in 2004. A total of 83% of infected flocks confirmed by laboratories were backyard chickens (56%) or ducks (27%). Outbreaks were concentrated in the Central, the southern part of the Northern and Eastern Regions of Thailand, which are wetlands, water reservoirs and dense poultry areas. More than 62 million birds were either killed by HPAI viruses or culled.[24]

Phylogenetic studies of the viral genome of H5N1 were carried out to compare and contrast different H5N1 strains from various times and places throughout Asia. The key role in influenza virus pathogenicity is the HA glycoprotein and proteolytic activation to take part in viral infectivity and dissemination. The first whole genome of the Thai avian influenza virus A (H5N1) — A/Chicken/Nakorn-Pathom/Thailand/CU-K2/04 — isolated from the Thai avian influenza epidemic during the early of 2004 was sequenced. Phylogenetic analyses were performed in comparison to avian influenza viruses from Hong Kong 1997 outbreaks and other H5N1 isolates reported during 2001–2004. Molecular characterization of the Thai avian influenza (H5N1) hemagglutinin gene revealed a common characteristic of a HPAI, which contained multiple basic amino acids at the cleavage site, a 20-codon deletion in the neuraminidase gene, a five-codon deletion in the NS gene, amantadine-resistant polymorphisms of the M2 and polymorphism of the PB2 genes.[25] In addition, a single amino acid substitution from Glutamic acid (E) to Lysine (K) at position 627 related to increased virus replication efficiency in mammals[26] was observed. Moreover, the HA and NA genes of the Thai avian influenza displayed high similarity to those of the viruses isolated from human cases during the same epidemic.[27] Additionally, after sequencing and comparing amino acids of hemaglutinin cleavage site sequence from various avian species with both wild and domestic birds in Thailand in 2003–2004, some variation among the isolates was found, from PQRERRRKKRto PQREKRRKKR, in openbill or PQRERKRKKR; in white peacock, kalij pheasant and crow. These viruses also exhibited a highly pathogenic characteristic, indicating that different amino acid sequences other than the sequence PQRERRRKKR could also be found in the HPAI (Figures 1 and 2).[28]

Spreading Ability of H5N1

Generally, human influenza is transmitted by inhalation of infectious droplets by direct contact or indirect contact, with self-inoculation onto the upper respiratory tract.[29] For human influenza A (H5N1) infections in Thailand to date, supporting data is consistent with bird-to-human, possible, environment-to-human and probable human-to-human transmission.[20] The exposure to live poultry within a week before the onset of illness was associated with disease in humans. Most patients have had a history of direct contact with poultry. For instance, gathering and preparing of diseased birds, handling fighting cocks and playing with poultry have all been concerned. Transmission to other mammals has been observed by feeding raw infected chickens to tigers and leopards in zoos in Thailand.[18,19] Several other modes of transmission are theoretically possible, given the survival of

(A)

HA gene cleavage site

```
                                                           330       340       350
A/Chicken/Mexico/31381/94(LPAI)                  ATGLRNVPQRE----TRGLFGAIAGF
A/chicken/Scotland/59(HPAI)                      ATGLRNVPQRK----KRGLFGAIAGF
A/Goose/Guangdong/1/96                           ATGLRNTPQRERRRKKRGLFGAIAGF
96-97  A/HongKong/156/97                         ATGLRNSPQRERRRKKRGLFGAIAGF
       A/HongKong/213/03                         ATGLRNSPQRERRRKKRGLFGAIAGF
       A/Ck/HK/SSP141/03                         ATGLRNSPQRERRRKKRGLFGAIAGF
03-04  A/chicken/Nakorn-Patom/Thailand/CU-K2/04  ATGLRNSPQRERRRKKRGLFGAIAGF
       A/tiger/Thailand/CU-T7/04                 ATGLRNSPQREKRRKKRGLFGAIAGF
       A/thailand/NK165/05                       ATGLRNSPQREKRRKKRGLFGAIAGF
05     A/chicken/Thailand/Kanchanaburi/CK-160/05 ATGLRNSPQREKRRKKRGLFGAIAGF
       A/chicken/Thailand/Nontaburi/CK-162/05    ATGLRNSPQREKRRKKRGLFGAIAGF
       A/quail/Thailand/Nakhonpathom/QA-161/05   ATGLRNSPQREKRRKKRGLFGAIAGF
                                                          ↑
```

(B)

NA gene 20 amino acid deletion

```
                                                             50        60        70        80
96-97  A/Goose/Guangdong/1/96                     SIQTGNQHQAEPCNQSIITYENNTWVNQTYVNISNTNFLTE
       A/HongKong/156/97                          IIQTWHPNQPEP------------------CNQSINFYTE
       A/HongKong/213/03                          SIQTGNQHQAEPCNQSIITYENNTWVNQTYVNISNTNFLTE
03-04  A/Ck/HK/SSP141/03                          SIHTGNQHQAEP------------------ISNTNFLAE
       A/tiger/Thailand/CU-T7/04                  SIHTGNQHKAEP------------------ISNTNLLTE
       A/chicken/Nakorn-Patom/Thailand/CU-K2/04   SIHTGNQHKAEP------------------ISNTNFLTE
       A/Thailand/NK165/05                        SIHTGNQQKAEP------------------ISNTNFLTE
05     A/chicken/Thailand/Kanchanaburi/CK-160/05  SIHTGNQQKAEP------------------ISNTNFLTE
       A/chicken/Thailand/Nontaburi/CK-162/05     SIHTGNQQKAEP------------------ISNTNFLTE
       A/quail/Thailand/NakhonPathom/QA-161/05    SIHTGNQQKAEP------------------ISNTNFLTE
```

(C)

NS gene 5 amino acid deletion

```
                                                           70        80        90
96-97  A/Goose/Guangdong/1/96                     EDILKSETNENLKIAIASSPAPRYITDMSI
       A/HongKong/156/97                          ERILEEESDEALKMTIASVPAPRYLTEMTL
       A/HK/213/03                                ERILEEESDEALKM-----PASRYLTDMTL
03-04  A/Ck/HK/SSP141/03                          ERILEEESDEALKM-----PASRYLTDMTL
       A/chicken/Nakorn-Patom/Thailand/CU-K2/04   ERILEEESDKALKM-----PASRYLTDMTL
       A/tiger/Chonburi/Thailand/CU-T7/04         ERILEEESDKALKM-----PASRYLTDMTL
       A/Thailand/NK165/05                        ERILEEESDKALKM-----PASRYLTDMTL
05     A/chicken/Thailand/Kanchanaburi/CK-160/05  ERILEEESDKALKM-----PASRYLTDMTL
       A/chicken/Thailand/Nontaburi/CK-162/05     ERILEEESDKALKM-----PASRYLTDMTL
       A/quail/Thailand/NakhonPathom/QA-161/05    ERILEEESDKALKM-----PASRYLTDMTL
```

(D)

PB2 gene amino acid change

```
                                                             620       630       640
96-97  A/Goose/Guangdong/1/96                     DTVQIIKLLPFAAAPPEPSRMQFSSLTVNVRG
       A/HongKong/156/97                          DTVQIIKLLPFAAAPPEQSRMQFSSLTVNVRG
       A/HK/213/03                                DTVQIIKLLPFAAAPPEQSRMQFSSLTVNVRG
03-04  A/Ck/HK/SSP141/2003                        DTVQIIKLLPFAAAPPEQSRMQFSSLTVNVRG
       A/chicken/Nakorn-Patom/Thailand/CU-K2/04   DTVQIIKLLPFAAAPPEQSRMQFSSLTVNVRG
       A/tiger/Chonburi/Thailand/CU-T7/04         DTVQIIKLLPFAAAPPKQSRMQFSSLTVNVRG
       A/Thailand/NK165/05                        DTVQVIKLLPFAAAPPKQNRMQFSSLTVNVRG
       A/quail/Thailand/NakhonPathom/QA-161/05    DTVQIIKLLPFAAAPPEQNRMQFSSLTVNVRG
05     A/chicken/Thailand/Nontaburi/CK-162/05     DTVQIIKLLPFAAAPPEQNRMQFSSLTVNVRG
       A/chicken/Thailand/Kanchanaburi/CK-160/05  DTVQIIKLLPFAAAPPEQNRMQFSSLTVNVRG
                                                                 ↑
```

Figure 1: Alignment comparisons of amino acid sequences of H5N1 avian influenza virus. (A) HA cleavage sites: Available sequences of viruses collected from 1996 through 2005 were compared which showed the alteration of amino acid Arginine (R) to Lysine (K) in virus of the year 2005 of Thailand. (B) NA stalk region: 20 amino acid residues have been deleted from the H5N1 influenza virus from Thailand during the year 2004–2005. (C) NS region: Five amino acid residues have been deleted from the gene. (D) PB2 region: Amino acid position 627 change from Glutamic acid (E) to Lysine (K) in mammal and human.

influenza A (H5N1) in the environment, such as oral ingestion of contaminated water during swimming, direct intranasal or conjunctival inoculation during exposure to water, contamination of hands from infected fomites and subsequent self-inoculation, contact poultry feces and contact patient samples. Human-to-human transmission of avian influenza has been suggested in several household clusters in Vietnam and in one case of apparent child-to-mother transmission in Thailand. On the contrary, serologic surveys in Vietnam and Thailand have not found evidence of asymptomatic infections among contacts.

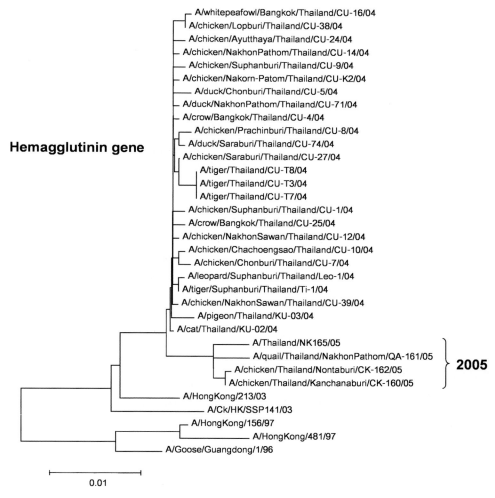

Figure 2: Phylogenetic analysis of hemagglutinin (HA) and neuraminidase (NA) genes of H5N1 avian influenza virus in Thailand.

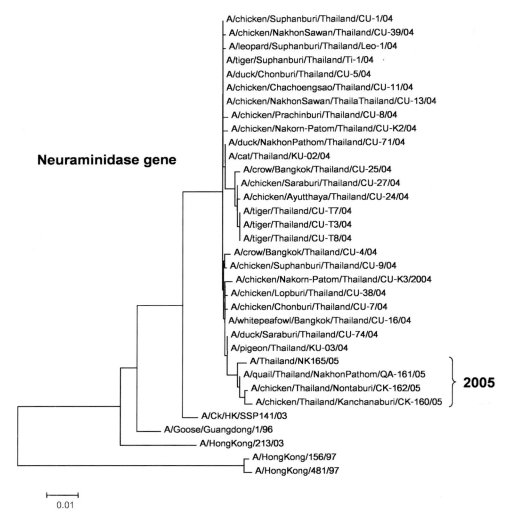

Figure 2: (*Continued*)

Clinical Manifestation

Incubation period: Normally, the incubation period from exposure to the source of infection to development of clinical symptoms is between two to four days.[30] Eight days are probable in some cases. During the outbreaks in 2004–2005, the incubation period was two to five days, with a range of maximum time of eight to 17 days.[31]

Clinical signs and symptoms: In general, there are four forms that are comprised of asymptomatic, mild URI, severe unexplained respiratory illness and multiple organ failure. All symptomatic patients have fever (temperature > 38°C). Minor symptoms are headache, myalgia, cough, sore throat, rhinorrhea, runny nose, vomit, diarrhea and eye infection (conjunctivitis).[16] Most of them have clinically apparent respiratory symptoms which develop into pneumonia. Radiographic findings include diffuse, multifocal, or patchy infiltrates, segmented or lobar consolidation. Severe cases have acute respiratory distress syndrome (ARDS) and multiple organ failure.[32]

Laboratory findings: Common laboratory findings showed leucopenia, particularly lymphopenia, thrombocytopenia and elevated serum transaminase value. In some patients, elevated creatinin levels were detected.

Atypical avian H5N1 influenza infection: An atypical case of avian influenza in humans has been reported in a patient who presented with diarrhea, without respiratory tract signs and symptoms.[17] From a recent study, de Jong et al.[33] reported two sibling Vietnamese patients presented with diarrhea without respiratory illness, followed by rapid progression to coma caused by acute encephalitis. Encephalitis and encephalopathy are unusual in humans who are infected with human influenza viruses. The clinical diagnosis of suspected H5N1 infected patients should focus not only on respiratory tract illness but also on unexplained death or other severe illness.

Mortality rate: Most of the patients died from severe progressive respiratory failure. The fatality rate among symptomatic patients who have been hospitalized is high. In Thailand, among 22 reported cases, there were 14 deaths (more than 60% mortality). The overall mortality rate of H5N1 infected reported cases until 2 February 2006 was 53.42%.[11]

Case Detection

The main clinical criteria to detect humans who are suspected of being infected with avian influenza (H5N1) infection have been reported by the US Centers for Disease Control and Prevention (CDC). A document is available on the CDC website (www.cdc.gov) and on the World Health Organization (WHO) website (www.who.int). This criterion is divided into three categories:

1. **Suspected case**
   A suspected patient is someone who has illness with fever higher or equal to 38°C, cough and/or sore throat. This patient has contact history within ten days of symptom onset to an affected area and close contact (within

one meter) with poultry, including poultry products and/or employment
in an occupation with potential exposure to HPAI. If the patient meets
both clinical and epidemical criteria, then collection of specimens and
submission for novel influenza virus testing are necessary.

2. **Probable case**

   A probable patient is the suspected patient who has been confirmed with
   primary laboratory diagnostics, for example immunofluorescence assay
   (IFA) and H5 monoclonal antibody, or shows no evidence of other possible causes.

3. **Confirmed case**

   A confirmed influenza A H5N1 patient is the patient who has detectable
   influenza A H5N1 by virus culture and/or has positive result of H5 virus
   by either reverse transcription polymerase chain reaction (RT-PCR) or
   four-fold titer increase of H5-specific antibody.

Specimen Collection

To ensure accurate results, it is necessary to collect specimens properly. Good
quality specimens should be collected early, during the start of illness. In
poultry, specimens that can be collected are carcasses, cloacal swabs, tracheal
swabs or stool. For humans, there are three main types of specimens, which
may be collected for viral diagnostics:[34]

1. **Respiratory specimens:**

   a. Sputum
   b. Oropharyngeal swabs
   c. Nasopharyngeal suction or wash

   The most appropriate human specimen is nasopharyngeal suction or
   wash collected by De le suction catheter. If the specimen is a throat swab,
   the sterile Dacron or Rayon swabs with plastic shafts should be used.
   Following specimen collection, the swabs should be placed immediately
   into sterile vials containing media.

2. **Blood components:** Collect whole blood in an EDTA tube and in a
   clotting tube.

3. **Autopsy specimens:** Appropriate tissues are central lung with segmental
   bronchi, right and left primary bronchi, trachea (proximal and distal) and
   representation pulmonary parenchyma from right and left lung. H5N1
   influenza A virus can infect as systemic disease, the virus can be isolated
   in many organs, for instance, liver, brain, spleen.

Laboratory Diagnostics

Several types of diagnostic tests are used for confirmation of H5N1 infection with the most appropriate specimen depending on the test. Each of the tests is described below.[35,36]

1. **Virus isolation**

    The gold standard for confirming that the virus is infectious, using eight- to 12-day-old embryonated egg or Mardin-Darby canine kidney (MDCK) cell.

    a. **Chicken embryo culture:** The virus is grown by inoculating influenza virus into the amniotic sac or allantoic sac of an embryonated egg. The amniotic or allantoic fluid is then used to detect influenza virus by hemagglutination (HA) and antigenic analysis (subtype) by hemagglutination inhibition (HAI).

    b. **Cell culture:** MDCK cells are the preferred cell line for culturing influenza viruses. Identification of virus isolates can usually be made on the basis of the type of cytopathic effect (CPE). Influenza viruses do not ordinarily induce CPE. Therefore, for final identification, HA or HAI are normally carried out.

2. **Immunofluorescense assay (IFA)**

    Immunofluorescense assay is used for the rapid detection of virus infections by the detection of virus-specific antibody. The basis of IFA technique makes use of a fluorescein-labeled antibody to stain specimens containing specific virus antigens, in order that the stained cells view the fluorescence under UV illumination. This method is highly dependent on the quality of the specimens, experience and requires highly skilled staff for the reading of the results.

3. **Hemagglutination and hemagglutination inhibition test**

    a. **Hemagglutination (HA) test:** The basis of this method is that influenza viruses possess the ability to agglutinate the erythrocytes of mammalian or avian species.

    b. **Hemagglutination inhibition (HAI) test:** If specimens have antibodies against the viral protein responsible for HA, it can prevent HA; this is the basis behind the HAI test. At present, the influenza virus can be divided into subtypes by using antisera specific to each of the different subtypes.

4. **Rapid antigen test**

This test is used to distinguish influenza A from other respiratory illnesses, but cannot identify into avian influenza A subtypes. Of note, there are commercial kits available and their use can provide results within 30 minutes.

5. **Molecular techniques**

Molecular techniques are based on the direct detection of viral genomes in the specimen. Reverse transcription polymerase chain reaction (RT-PCR) and real-time RT-PCR are the most commonly used methods for the detection of avian influenza virus in the present day.[37] The Center of Excellence in Viral Hepatitis Research, Faculty of Medicine, Chulalongkorn University developed one-step multiplex RT-PCR and multiplex real-time RT-PCR for rapid detection of HA, NA and M genes[38,39] and developed the rapid method for discriminating between HPAI and LPAI strain by using melting curve analysis PCR.[40]

Avian Influenza Management

Since this disease is originated from a virus, it cannot be cured by antibiotics. The treatment is similar to other respiratory diseases caused by viral infection. At the present time, there are two groups of drug against influenza viruses.

Adamantane derivative: Adamantane derivative is an M2 protein ion channel inhibitor containing amantadine and rimantadine. This drug should be provided within two to four days of illness onset for a 70%–90% efficacy in preventing and treating type A influenza only. The use of M2 inhibitors, particularly for treatment, is likely to lead to the emergence and spread of drug-resistant influenza viruses. Recently, WHO has reported H5N1 virus resistance to amantadine and rimantadine.[41]

Neuraminidase inhibitor: The neuraminidase inhibitors, Zanamivir and Oseltamivir, are superior to M2 inhibitors with regards to serious side effects. Zanamivir comes in the form of an inhaled powder while Oseltamivir is the first orally active antiviral drug. Currently, there have been no reports of Zanamivir-resistant viruses, although there is an emergence of Oseltamivir-resistant ones. The hypothesis is that the chemical structure of Oseltamivir could facilitate the development of resistant mutations that would permit neuraminidase to function, allowing drug-resistant viruses to survive and propagate. Molecular analyses of amino acids of neuraminidase protein show the rotation at E276 and bond with R224 to form the side chain of

Oseltamivir. The mutations R292K, N294S and H274Y inhibit this rotation and prevent the chain from forming, resulting in resistance to Oseltamivir. In contrast, the binding of Zanamivir does not require any re-orientation of amino acids.[41,42]

Avian Influenza Vaccine

To date, the efficacious H5N1 vaccine is still not available to humans. In practice, the currently available human influenza vaccine cannot protect against the avian influenza subtype H5N1. As the influenza virus is an RNA virus, the vaccine can change easily to accommodate new strains, which normally results in a vaccine component change every year. Some subtypes of avian influenza vaccine are currently available (including the H5 subtype vaccine available in poultry), but the evidence of cross-protection is questionable. The advantages of vaccination include poultry protection from illness and death as well as reduction of the spread of virus. In a different way, the vaccine is incapable of 100% protection against the virus, resulting in the increasing risk of viral exposure to farmers. Moreover, the report about the effect of vaccine in the evolution of Mexican lineage H5N2 avian influenza showed the viruses isolated after the introduction of vaccine belonged to sublineages separate from the vaccine's sublineage which indicates multi-lineage antigenic drift, and the persistence of the virus in the field that is likely aided by its large antigenic difference from the vaccine strain.[43]

Recommendation for People who Reside in Outbreak Areas[44]

General recommendations:
1. Avoid direct contact with poultry, any part of them, feces and carcasses.
2. Keep the body healthy.
3. Wash hands and body with soap and water for 15–20 seconds after contact with contaminated surfaces, feces and secretion of poultry.
4. See a doctor immediately if body temperature raises equal or more than 38°C, cough and/or sore throat.
5. Take the precaution in affected regions where avian influenza H5N1 has been confirmed.

Transporter recommendations:
1. Do not move the poultry when there is an outbreak in the poultry population.
2. Clean vehicles and cages with detergent.

3. Do not purchase poultry from infected farms.
4. Take appropriate personal protection, clean the body with soap and change into a new set of clothes after work.

Farm workers recommendations:

1. Destroy all infected poultry and carcasses and clean the environmental area.
2. Protect against other animals, such as birds and rodents, from entering chicken housing.
3. Farm workers who are in close contact with infected animals or are exposed to contaminated farms should have personal protective suits, such as surgical gowns with long cuffed sleeves, plus impermeable aprons, masks, goggles, gloves and boots.

Laboratory and healthcare workers recommendations:
The laboratory and healthcare workers should be reminded of the importance of handling and transporting specimens of the suspected infection. Laboratory workers have to perform the testing under biosafety (category III) or BSL3 containment laboratory conditions for infectious materials in order to prevent the spread of virus to other healthcare or laboratory workers. Handling of uninfected products for testing using polymerase chain reaction (PCR) methods come under biosafety level 2 (BSL2).

Consumer recommendations:

1. Avoid visiting live animal markets and poultry farms.
2. Purchase only chicken and chicken products from a standardized shop.
3. Use separate kitchen utensils for raw and cooked meats.
4. Poultry products should be cooked until all parts reach an internal temperature of more than 70°C.
5. Wash hands with detergent after touching any poultry products.

Conclusion

Avian influenza viruses are normally species-specific and circulate in birds. Since 1997, there have been several outbreaks of highly pathogenic avian influenza virus in poultry flocks and they have crossed the species barrier to infect humans. Resulting patients have severe symptoms and infection which can lead to death. Southeast Asia is the origin of this outbreak. To date, influenza H5N1 strains that have circulated through to Eurasia are the strain that was first isolated in Hong Kong in 1997. It seems that this virus have been able to spread around the world within a year of initial detection. The outbreak of H5N1 is unlikely to be the last in the near future. We must be prepared and take preventive measures in the event of a pandemic, through extensive influenza surveillance, vaccine development and production, antiviral therapy and influenza-related research.

Acknowledgments

The studies were supported by the Thailand Research Fund (Senior Research Scholar); Royal Golden Jubilee PhD Program; Center of Excellence in Viral Hepatitis Research, Chulalongkorn University; The Department of Livestock Development, National Institute of Animal Health, Bangkok, Thailand; and The Virology Unit, Faculty of Veterinary Science, Chulalongkorn University.

References

1. Turner D, Wailoo A, Nicholson K, Cooper N, Sutton A, Abrams K. Systematic review and economic decision modelling for the prevention and treatment of influenza A and B. *Health Technol Assess* 2003;7(iii–iv, xi–xiii):1–170.
2. Nicholson KG, Wood JM, Zambon M. Influenza. *Lancet* 2003;362:1733–1745.
3. Lamb RA, Krug RM. *Orthomyxoviridae*: the viruses and their replication. In: *Fields Virology*, 4th ed. (eds.) Knipe DM, Howley PM, Lippincott Williams & Wilkins, Philadelphia, 2001, pp. 725–770.
4. Fouchier RA, Munster V, Wallensten A, Bestebroer TM, Herfst S, Smith D, Rimmelzwaan GF, Olsen B, Osterhaus AD. Characterization of a novel influenza A virus hemagglutinin subtype (H16) obtained from black-headed gulls. *J Virol* 2005;79:2814–2822.
5. Gamblin SJ, Haire LF, Russell RJ, Stevens DJ, Xiao B, Ha Y, Vasisht N, Steinhauer DA, Daniels RS, Elliot A, Wiley DC, Skehel JJ. The structure and receptor binding properties of the 1918 influenza hemagglutinin. *Science* 2004;303:1838–1842.
6. Claas EC, Osterhaus AD, van Beek R, De Jong JC, Rimmelzwaan GF, Senne DA, Krauss S, Shortridge KF, Webster RG. Human influenza A H5N1 virus related to a highly pathogenic avian influenza virus. *Lancet* 1998;351:472–477.
7. Nicholson KG, Wood JM, Zambon M. Influenza. *Lancet* 2003;362:1733–1745.
8. Webster RG, Geraci J, Petursson G, Skirnisson K. Conjunctivitis in human beings caused by influenza A virus of seals. *N Engl J Med* 1981;304:911.
9. Fouchier RAM. *Avian Influenza, Human — Netherlands (09): Fatal Case*, Promed 13 April 2003. Accessed from website http://www.promedmail.org (Archive No. 20030419.0959).

10. World Organization for Animal Health. *Update on Avian Influenza in Animals (Type H5)*. [Updated 6 February 2006]. Available from http://www.oie.int/downld/AVIAN%20INFLUENZA/A_AI-Asia.htm

11. World Health Organization. *Cumulative Number of Confirmed Human Cases of Avian Influenza A/(H5N1) Reported to WHO*. [Updated 2 February 2006]. Available from http://www.who.int/csr/disease/avian_influenza/country/cases_table_2006_02_02/en/index.html

12. Li KS, Guan Y, Wang J, Smith GJ, Xu KM, Duan L, Rahardjo AP, Puthavathana P, Buranathai C, Nguyen TD, Estoepangestie AT, Chaisingh A, Auewarakul P, Long HT, Hanh NT, Webby RJ, Poon LL, Chen H, Shortridge KF, Yuen KY, Webster RG, Peiris JS. Genesis of a highly pathogenic and potentially pandemic H5N1 influenza virus in eastern Asia. *Nature* 2004;430:209–213.

13. World Health Organization. *H5N1 Avian Influenza: Timeline*. [Updated 28 October 2005]. Available from http://www.who.int/csr/disease/avian_influenza/Timeline_28_10a.pdf

14. Kuiken T, Rimmelzwaan G, van Riel D, van Amerongen G, Baars M, Fouchier R, Osterhaus A. Avian H5N1 influenza in cats. *Science* 2004;306:241.

15. Liu J, Xiao H, Lei F, Zhu Q, Qin K, Zhang XW, Zhang XL, Zhao D, Wang G, Feng Y, Ma J, Liu W, Wang J, Gao GF. Highly pathogenic H5N1 influenza virus infection in migratory birds. *Science* 2005;309:1206.

16. Chotpitayasunondh T, Ungchusak K, Hanshaoworakul W, Chunsuthiwat S, Sawanpanyalert P, Kijphati R, Lochindarat S, Srisan P, Suwan P, Osotthanakorn Y, Anantasetagoon T, Kanjanawasri S, Tanupattarachai S, Weerakul J, Chaiwirattana R, Maneerattanaporn M, Poolsavathitikool R, Chokephaibulkit K, Apisarnthanarak A, Dowell SF. Human disease from influenza A (H5N1), Thailand, 2004. *Emerg Infect Dis* 2005;11:201–209.

17. Apisarnthanarak A, Kitphati R, Thongphubeth K, Patoomanunt P, Anthanont P, Auwanit W, Thawatsupha P, Chittaganpitch M, Saeng-Aroon S, Waicharoen S, Apisarnthanarak P, Storch GA, Mundy LM, Fraser VJ. Atypical avian influenza (H5N1). *Emerg Infect Dis* 2004;10:1321–1324.

18. Keawcharoen J, Oraveerakul K, Kuiken T, Fouchier RA, Amonsin A, Payungporn S, Noppornpanth S, Wattanodorn S, Theambooniers A, Tantilertcharoen R, Pattanarangsan R, Arya N, Ratanakorn P, Osterhaus DM, Poovorawan Y. Avian influenza H5N1 in tigers and leopards. *Emerg Infect Dis* 2004;10:2189–2191.

19. Thanawongnuwech R, Amonsin A, Tantilertcharoen R, Damrongwatanapokin S, Theamboonlers A, Payungporn S, Nanthapornphiphat K, Ratanamungklanon S, Tunak E, Songserm T, Vivatthanavanich V, Lekdumrongsak T, Kesdangsakonwut S, Tunhikorn S, Poovorawan Y. Probable tiger-to-tiger transmission of avian influenza H5N1. *Emerg Infect Dis* 2005;11:699–701.

20. Ungchusak K, Auewarakul P, Dowell SF, Kitphati R, Auwanit W, Puthavathana P, Uiprasertkul M, Boonnak K, Pittayawonganon C, Cox NJ,

Zaki SR, Thawatsupha P, Chittaganpitch M, Khontong R, Simmerman JM, Chunsutthiwat S. Probable person-to-person transmission of avian influenza A (H5N1). *N Engl J Med* 2005;352:333–340.

21. World Health Organization Global Influenza Program Surveillance Network. Evolution of H5N1 avian influenza viruses in Asia. *Emerg Infect Dis* 2005;11:1515–1521.

22. Marshall M. *Avian Influenza, Human — Eurasia (43): Iraq, Turkey*, Promed 31 January 2006. Accessed from website http://www.promedmail.org (Archive No. 20060131.0317).

23. Webster RG, Bean WJ, Gorman OT, Chambers TM, Kawaoka Y. Evolution and ecology of influenza A viruses. *Microbiol Rev* 1992;56:152–179.

24. Tiensin T. Highly pathogenic avian influenza H5N1, Thailand, 2004. *Emerg Infect Dis* 2005;11:1664–1672.

25. Viseshakul N, Thanawongnuwech R, Amonsin A, Suradhat S, Payungporn S, Keawchareon J, Oraveerakul K, Wongyanin P, Plitkul S, Theamboonlers A, Poovorawan Y. The genome sequence analysis of H5N1 avian influenza A virus isolated from the outbreak among poultry populations in Thailand. *Virology* 2004;328:169–176.

26. Shinya K, Hamm S, Hatta M, Ito H, Ito T, Kawaoka Y. PB2 amino acid at position 627 affects replicative efficiency, but not cell tropism, of Hong Kong H5N1 influenza A viruses in mice. *Virology* 2004;320:258–266.

27. Puthavathana P, Auewarakul P, Charoenying PC, Sangsiriwut K, Pooruk P, Boonnak K, Khanyok R, Thawachsupa P, Kijphati R, Sawanpanyalert P. Molecular characterization of the complete genome of human influenza H5N1 virus isolates from Thailand. *J Gen Virol* 2005;86:423–433.

28. Keawcharoen J, Amonsin A, Oraveerakul K, Wattanodorn S, Papravasit T, Karnda S, Lekakul K, Pattanarangsan R, Noppornpanth S, Fouchier RA, Osterhaus AD, Payungporn S, Theamboonlers A, Poovorawan Y. Characterization of the hemagglutinin and neuraminidase genes of recent influenza virus isolates from different avian species in Thailand. *Acta Virol* 2005;49:277–280.

29. Bridges CB, Kuehnert MJ, Hall CB. Transmission of influenza: implications for control in health care settings. *Clin Infect Dis* 2003;37:1094–1101.

30. Yuen KY, Chan PK, Peiris M, *et al.* Clinical features and rapid viral diagnosis of human disease associated with avian influenza A H5N1 virus. *Lancet* 1998;351:467–471.

31. The Writing Committee of the World Health Organization (WHO) Consultation on Human Influenza A/H5. Current concepts: avian influenza A (H5N1) infection in humans. *N Engl J Med* 2005;353:1374–1385.

32. Tran TH, Nguyen TL, Nguyen TD, Luong TS, Pham PM, Nguyen VC, Pham TS, Vo CD, Le TQ, Ngo TT, Dao BK, Le PP, Nguyen TT, Hoang TL, Cao VT, Le TG, Nguyen DT, Le HN, Nguyen KT, Le HS, Le VT, Christiane D, Tran TT, Menno de J, Schultsz C, Cheng P, Lim W, Horby P, Farrar J. World Health Organization

International Avian Influenza Investigative Team. Avian influenza A (H5N1) in 10 patients in Vietnam. *N Engl J Med* 2004;350:1179–1188.

33. de Jong MD, Bach VC, Phan TQ, Vo MH, Tran TT, Nguyen BH, Beld M, Le TP, Truong HK, Nguyen VV, Tran TH, Do QH, Farrar J. Fatal avian influenza A (H5N1) in a child presenting with diarrhea followed by coma. *N Engl J Med* 2005;352:686–691.

34. United States Department of Health and Human Services. *HHS Pandemic Influenza Plan, Part 2 Public Health Guidance for State and Local Partners, Supplement 2 Laboratory Diagnostics, S2-1-30.* Available from http://www.hhs.gov/pandemicflu/plan/pdf/HHSPandemicInfluenzaPlan.pdf

35. CDC: Department of Health and Human Service. *Influenza (Flu): Laboratory Diagnostic Procedure for Influenza.* Available from http://www.cdc.gov/flu/professionals/labdiagnosis.htm

36. WHO, Geneva. *Manual on Animal Influenza Diagnosis and Surveillance* (WHO/CDS/CSR/NCS/2002.2). Available from http://www.who.int/csr/resources/publications/ influenza/ en/ whocdscsmcs2002.5.pdf

37. Ellos JS, Zambon MC. Molecular diagnosis of influenza. *Rev Med Virol* 2002;12:375–389.

38. Payungporn S, Phakdeewirot P, Chutinimitkul S, Theamboonlers A, Keawcharoen J, Oraveerakul K, Amonsin A, Poovorawan Y. Single-step multiplex reverse transcription-polymerase chain reaction (RT-PCR) for influenza A virus subtype H5N1 detection. *Viral Immunol* 2004;17:588–593.

39. Payungporn S, Chutinimitkul S, Chaisingh A, Damrongwantanapokin S, Buranathai C, Amonsin A, *et al.* Single step multiplex real-time RT-PCR for H5N1 influenza A virus detection. *J Virol Methods* 2006;131:143–147.

40. Payungporn S, Chutinimitkul S, Chaisingh A, Damrongwantanapokin S, Nuansrichay B, Pinyochon W, Amonsin A, Donis RO, Theamboonlers A, Poovorawan Y. Discrimination between highly and low pathogenic subtype H5 avian influenza A viruses by melting curve analysis real-time PCR. *Emerge Infect Dis*, 2006 (accepted).

41. United States Department of Health and Human Services. *HHS Pandemic Influenza Plan, Part 2 Public Health Guidance for State and Local Partners, Supplement 7 Antiviral Drug Distribution and Use, S7-1-19.*

42. Moscona A. Oseltamivir resistance-disabling our influenza defenses. *N Engl J Med* 2005;355:2633–2636.

43. Lee CW, Senne DA, Suarez DL. Effect of vaccine use in the evolution of Mexican lineage H5N2 avian influenza virus. *J Virol* 2004;78:8372–8381.

44. United States Department of Health and Human Services. *HHS Pandemic Influenza Plan, Part 2 Public Health Guidance for State and Local Partners, Supplement 4 Recommendations for Infection Control, S4-6-22.*

5

Epidemiology and Risk Factors for Avian Influenza

Thana Khawcharoenporn, Linda M. Mundy and Anucha Apisarnthanarak

Introduction

There were three notable influenza pandemics during the 20th century, each attributable to the emergence of a novel influenza A virus. For the emergence of new strains, one of at least two possible events must occur. The proximity of two viruses permit genetic reassortment as a single viral strain with novel viral surface proteins. The major global implication of such reassortment is that there is little population-based immunity to this new virus (Table 1). Alternatively, the virus may mutate in response to adaptation pressure to facilitate replication and, hence, have increased pathogenicity. In 1918, the Spanish influenza virus was the first to emerge. It was a highly virulent, swinelike H1N1 subtype influenza A virus that efficiently spread worldwide and resulted in an estimated 50 million human deaths.[1] The second pandemic occurred in 1957 when a new H2N2 influenza virus emerged in several Asian countries. This Asian influenza virus was associated with an estimated one million human deaths. Eleven years later, in 1968, the H2N2 subtype Asian influenza virus was replaced by a new human H3N2 strain. This strain, called the Hong Kong influenza virus, was the cause of the third 20th century influenza pandemic, associated with an estimated one million human deaths, and geographically targeted to Asia-Pacific countries.[2]

Table 1: Influenza A viruses associated with the 20th century pandemics.

Pandemic year	Influenza A virus	Reassortment
1918	H1N1	None (avian origin)
1957	H2N2, Asian	Human-avian
1968	H3N2, Hong Kong	Human-avian

In the fall of 1997, the first avian influenza A (H5N1) virus outbreak occurred. The virus had previously been confined to avian species and was isolated from humans in Hong Kong. There was a 33% human case fatality rate (six deaths among 18 clinically documented cases) associated with the outbreak, during which a mandated territory-wide slaughter of more than 1.5 million chickens ensued.[3] This costly intervention, with huge economic loss to the poultry business in Hong Kong, has been attributed to thwarting disease transmission and additional cases.[3] In February 2003, two additional patients with H5N1 were reported in Hong Kong, one of whom died. At almost the same time, there was a massive outbreak of another highly pathogenic avian influenza A virus — H7N7 subtype in commercial poultry farms in the Netherlands. Although the risk of human transmission of the virus was initially thought to be low, an outbreak investigation revealed the transmission of H7N7 to 85 people. The H7N7 cases presented with conjunctivitis — an influenza-like illness. Additionally, H7N7 infection was detected at least 255 chicken farms from which mandatory slaughter of an estimated 30 million chickens (28% of the chicken population in the Netherlands) ensued with an estimated loss of €284 million (US$338 million) to the Dutch economy million).[4] During late 2003 and early 2004, there were reports of large outbreaks of H5N1 among poultry throughout Asia including South Korea, Japan, Indonesia, Vietnam, Thailand, Laos, Cambodia and China. More than 120 million poultry died or were destroyed as part of the massive control program, with high impact on the Asia-Pacific economies. The outbreaks of H5N1 reappeared again in July 2003 in five Asian countries, with human cases identified in Vietnam and Thailand.[5,6] The cumulative number of virologically confirmed human cases of avian influenza (H5N1) reported to the World Health Organization (WHO) between December 2003 and January 2006 was 152 — with a 55% ($n = 83$) case fatality rate.[7]

To date, it is not clear whether the current avian influenza (H5N1) strain is capable of adapting to humans and efficiently inducing human-to-human transmission in populations at large. Nonetheless, two features of the H5N1 outbreaks enhance global concerns for a pandemic — the predominance of infections in children and young adults and the high mortality rates reported in these small outbreaks. A number of genetic changes resembling the changes of the 1918 pandemic influenza virus have been found in recently circulating, highly pathogenic avian influenza (H5N1) viruses.[8] In addition, the current H5N1 viruses have undergone antigenic drift, especially for the hemagglutinin antigens, the host range for the viruses has expanded, and temporally there seems to be an incremental rise in mortality rates for human cases.[9] Together, these findings suggest the potential of H5N1 viruses as the point source of the next influenza pandemic.

Epidemiology

Human infections with influenza A viruses associated with 20th century pandemics. The genetic characteristics of the 1918 H1N1 influenza virus provide an explanatory framework for the evolution of an influenza virus to a pandemic virus. In one study, the genomic RNA of the 1918 virus was reconstructed from archived formalin-fixed lung autopsy tissue of an Alaskan influenza victim to study the properties associated with its extraordinary virulence.[1] The study revealed that the 1918 H1N1 influenza virus could replicate in the absence of trypsin, suggesting neuraminidase (NA)-facilitated hemagglutinin (HA) cleavage not found in contemporary human influenza viruses. The reconstructed virus also caused death in mice and displayed a high growth phenotype in human bronchial epithelial cells.[1] These findings may be relevant to the high pathogenic activity noted in human cases. In terms of molecular analysis, the polymerase protein sequences from the 1918 H1N1 virus differed from avian consensus sequences at only ten amino acids, suggesting that the virus might have originated from an avian influenza virus. However, the difference in the ten amino acid changes may have contributed to human adaptation and made the 1918 virus more transmissible to humans than other avian influenza viruses.[8]

The genetic sequences of the current strain of influenza virus, 1997 Hong Kong H5N1 and 2004 Vietnam H5N1, have been compared to the 1918 H1N1 virus (Table 2). Several viral isolates of the two origins contained only one of the ten amino acid changes of the 1918 virus.[8] These findings may partially explain why the H5N1 viruses did not cause a human influenza pandemic. Additive genetic changes would be needed over time before these viruses could spread efficiently from person to person as historically noted during the 1918 pandemic.[10]

Table 2: Comparisons of the 1918 influenza virus with the H5N1 viruses.

Virus	Genetic differences	Reassortment	Host range
1918 H1N1	Ten amino acid changes from avian influenza	None	Human
1997 Hong Kong H5N1	Genotype Z, Clade 3	Quail H9N2 virus and a teal H6N1 virus	Human and avian species
2004 Vietnam H5N1	Genotype Z, Clade 1	No data	Human and avian species
2004 Thailand H5N1	Genotype Z, Clade 1	No data	Human, avian species, pig, tiger, leopard, cat

Note: Avian species = Species of birds including chickens, ducks, geese, swans and waterfowls.

Asymptomatic infection and seropositivity. In 1997, a study conducted during the H5N1 outbreak in Hong Kong demonstrated that asymptomatic healthcare workers who were exposed to H5N1 case patients had a significantly higher seroprevalence of H5 antibody than those who were not exposed to the patients.[3] Three percent of poultry cullers were reported to have seroconversion of H5 antibody in Hong Kong during 1997, as well as 1% of poultry cullers in Indonesia in 2005.[11] Another ongoing study involving the screening for H5 antibody in 120 hospitalized adults with severe community acquired pneumonia patients in Thailand revealed that one patient who had a history of exposure to poultry did have seropositivity for H5N1 virus (unpublished data). These data suggest that asymptomatic hosts can develop H5N1 antibody after exposure to infected poultry.

Host range. In general, most avian strains of the influenza viruses are of low pathogenicity. The avian influenza strains vary greatly in genetic composition, owing to 16 HAs (H1 through H16) and nine NAs (N1 through N9). The viruses have spread into domestic poultry, caused silent infection in domestic ducks in Southern China and had a lower lethal dose in mammalian animal models of infection.[12] Although the avian strains are widespread in migratory birds and waterfowls, over the past eight years only three subtypes have caused human respiratory infection (H1N1, H2N2 and H3N2), suggesting some level of host specificity. The most current strain of influenza A virus, H5N1, has been reported to have an extended host range. In 2003, the H5N1 virus was isolated from diseased pigs on farms in Southern China, marking the first documented natural infection of pigs with any viruses of the H5 subtype.[13] Some wild migratory birds in Mongolia and Russia and migratory swans in Croatia have been reported to directly transmit H5N1 to domestic poultry.[14] Domestic birds may become infected with the virus through direct contact with infected waterfowls or other infected poultry, or through contact with surfaces (such as dirt or cages) or materials (such as water or feed) that have been contaminated with the virus.[15] Tigers (*Panthera tigris*) and leopards (*Panthera pardus*) in a zoo in Thailand had been infected with the H5N1 viruses and died after they were fed raw chicken carcasses that were possibly contaminated with H5N1 viruses.[16] Additionally, a study revealed that cats were infected with H5N1 virus by horizontal transmission and by ingestion of virus-contaminated birds.[17] Moreover, the threat of H5N1 transmission via international air travel was spotlighted when the viruses were isolated from Crested Hawk-Eagles (*Spizaetus nipalensis*) smuggled into Europe from Thailand.[18] Together, these findings emphasize that the host range of H5N1 viruses is broad compared to previously characterized influenza A viruses that were able to infect humans.

Human infections with avian influenza H5N1 associated with outbreaks over the past decade. The three major outbreaks of H5N1 viruses — in Hong Kong, Vietnam and Thailand, are exemplary of viral transmission attributable to genetic reassortment of avian and human influenza viruses. In Hong Kong, the first case of H5N1 infection identified in humans occurred in May 1997. No additional cases were reported for six months, after which an additional 17 cases in two months were identified, defining the second wave of the epidemic.[3] Among these 18 infected cases, ten were female and eight were ≤12 years of age. Epidemiologic and molecular evidence suggests that poultry was the source of the H5N1 outbreak. Large-scale outbreaks had occurred in chicken farms in the northwestern part of Hong Kong in March and April 1997, just before the first human case was identified and reported. Then high rates of infection again occurred in poultry in October, November and December of the same year, shortly before the second wave of the epidemic in humans.[3] The genetic sequencing data and the temporal relationship between avian and human outbreaks strongly suggest that direct chicken-to-human cross-species transmission of the virus occurred without the involvement of an intermediate host. Several molecular epidemiologic studies were conducted to trace the origin of this lethal H5N1 strain. Current evidence suggests that the Hong Kong 1997 H5N1 strain included reassortants from a co-circulating quail H9N2 virus and a teal H6N1 virus.[3]

In Vietnam, the outbreak of H5N1 virus occurred in ten patients between December 2003 and January 2004.[5] Four were female, the mean age was

13.7 years, and the patients were from both rural and urban parts of Vietnam. There was clear evidence of either direct handling of poultry (chickens or ducks) or exposure to sick poultry in the week before the onset of illnesses in eight patients. The available laboratory diagnostic information confirmed bird-to-human transmission, but there is currently not enough information to rule out limited human-to-human transmission.[5]

In Thailand, the H5N1 virus epidemic in poultry took place during two distinct time periods, January to May 2004 and July to December 2004. The latter period was temporally related to the known peak seasonal variation of human influenza in Thailand (June through August). According to the Thailand Department of Livestock, poultry populations in 1417 villages in 60 of 76 provinces were affected by H5N1 viruses in 2004, with laboratory confirmation of infection in 83% of ill flocks (56% backyard chickens and 27% ducks).[19] Outbreaks were concentrated in the southern part of the Northern, Central and Eastern regions of Thailand, which comprise wetlands, water reservoirs and areas with dense poultry (Figure 1). More than 62 million birds were either killed by highly pathogenic avian influenza (HPAI) viruses or culled.[19] The high numbers of HPAI cases detected coincided with low temperatures in Thailand during the first period of the epidemic, when wild birds from central and northern Asia migrated into Thailand. Together, the seasonal conditions and bird migration may have contributed to the introduction of HPAI virus, while the lower temperatures that supports survival of H5N1 viruses in the environment may have facilitated transmission. In addition, several festivals, which are associated with raising, selling and transporting poultry, traditionally occur, and did occur, around the end of the 2004 calendar year.[19]

There were 12 confirmed human cases of avian influenza H5N1 from January through March 2004 in Thailand. The median age was 12 years, with seven children <14 years of age and five adults. All patients resided in a village with a high rate of chicken deaths. Nine cases lived in houses with backyard chickens that died unexpectedly and eight reported direct contact with dead chickens. Notably, there were no suspected or confirmed avian influenza H5N1 cases among Thai health personnel.[6] The molecular characterization of the 12 viral isolates revealed that amino acid residues at the receptor-binding site of the viruses were similar to those of the chicken virus and other H5N1 viruses from Hong Kong. In addition, all genomic segments of the Thailand viruses clustered with the recently described genotype Z.[20] However, the Thailand viruses contained more avian-specific residues than the 1997 Hong Kong H5N1 viruses, suggesting that the virus may have adapted to allow a more efficient spread in avian species.[20]

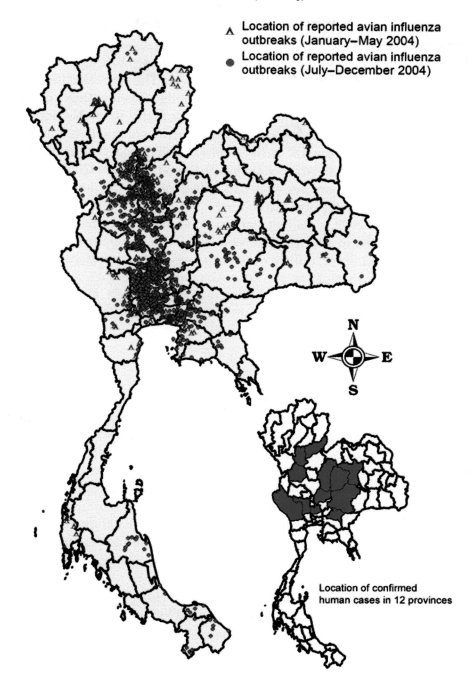

Figure 1: Distribution of reported highly pathogenic avian influenza H5N1 outbreaks in villages in Thailand, January–May 2004 (188 villages of 193 flocks) and July–December 2004 (1243 villages of 1492 flocks). *Source*: *Emerging Infectious Diseases Journal*, Vol. 11, No. 11, pp. 1664–1672, 2005 (published by the Centers for Disease Control and Prevention, USA).[19]

Avian influenza A viruses other than the H5N1 outbreak strains have also been reported. Low pathogenic avian influenza A, subtype H9N2, infection was confirmed in two children in China and Hong Kong in 1999 and resulted in uncomplicated influenza-like illnesses. The source of the viruses was unknown, but evidence suggested that poultry was the source of infection and bird-to-human transmission was implicated.[21] In the Netherlands, the HPAI influenza A subtype H7N7 caused acute conjunctivitis in a veterinarian who visited several farms with HPAI-infected poultry flocks in March 2003. By June 2003, there were 89 confirmed cases of H7N7 infection, most of whom were workers who had culled poultry. All isolated H7N7 viruses at that time were of avian origin.[4]

In November 2003, a patient with serious underlying medical conditions was admitted to a hospital in New York with respiratory symptoms, after which H7N2 avian influenza A virus was isolated and attributed to infection.[21] In February 2004, an outbreak of avian influenza A H7N3 was reported in poultry in the Fraser Valley region of Canada, along with two confirmed human cases, both of whom had extensive exposure to poultry.[22]

Risk Factors

The main route of human transmission of avian influenza viruses is direct contact with infected poultry or surfaces and objects contaminated with infected poultry's fecal material. To date, most human cases have occurred in either rural geographic regions or where households keep small poultry flocks that occupy household space or children's play areas.[11] As infected birds excrete and shed large quantities of virus, human exposure to infected bird droppings or to environments contaminated by avian influenza viruses are numerous. In addition, many households in Asia-Pacific countries economically depend on the family's poultry business and ill poultry may not be readily recognized in the early disease phases, thus augmenting viral exposure to other animals and to humans.

During the 1997 H5N1 influenza outbreak in Hong Kong, a case-control study was conducted of 15 patients hospitalized for H5N1 disease. Exposure to live poultry before the onset of illness was significantly associated with the disease, whereas travel, preparation of and ingestion of poultry products were not associated risks.[3]

During the 2004 outbreak in Vietnam, direct handling of poultry (chickens or ducks) or exposure to sick poultry in the week before the onset of illnesses were risk factors for infection.[5] A case report of H5N1 infection in a child suggested that contact with canal water where infected domestic ducks swam was the point source of exposure.[23]

In Thailand, the risk of H5N1 infection was evaluated during the 2004 outbreak. Direct contact with dead chickens, residence in a village with a high proportion of chicken deaths and residence in a home where backyard chickens died unexpectedly were all associated with H5N1 infection.[6]

Recommendations for people infected with avian influenza H5N1 infection have been developed by The Writing Committee of the World Health Organization (WHO) Consultation on Human Influenza A/H5.[11] For countries and territories where H5N1 viruses have been identified as a cause of illness in human or animal populations such as Hong Kong, Vietnam, Thailand, China and Cambodia, the following exposure may put a person at risk of H5N1 infection during the seven to 14 days antecedent to the onset of symptoms:

1. Contact (within one meter) with live or dead domestic fowl (including ducks) and wild birds.
2. Exposure to settings in which domestic fowl were confined or had been confined in the previous six weeks.
3. Unprotected contact [within touching or speaking distance (one meter)] with a person for whom the diagnosis of influenza A (H5N1) is confirmed or under consideration.
4. Unprotected contact [within touching or speaking distance (one meter)] with a person who had an unexplained acute respiratory illness that later resulted in severe pneumonia and death.
5. Occupational exposure in a domestic fowl worker, worker in a domestic fowl processing plant, domestic fowl culler (catching, bagging or transporting birds, or disposing of dead birds), worker in a live animal market, chef working with live or recently killed domestic fowl, dealer or trader in pet birds, healthcare worker or a worker in a laboratory processing samples possibly containing influenza A (H5N1) virus.

For countries and territories where H5N1 viruses have not been identified as a cause of illness in human or animal populations, the following exposure may put a person at risk of H5N1 infection during the seven to 14 days before the onset of symptoms:

1. Close contact with an ill traveler from one of the areas with known influenza A (H5N1) activity.
2. History of travel to a country or territory with reported avian influenza activity due to influenza A (H5N1) in the animal population and living

in an area in which there are reported deaths of domestic fowl with one or more of the following:

- Contact (within one meter) with live or dead domestic fowl (including ducks) or wild birds in any setting.
- Exposure to settings in which domestic fowl were confined or had been confined in the previous six weeks.
- Contact [within touching or speaking distance (one meter)] with a confirmed case patient of influenza A (H5N1).
- Contact [within touching or speaking distance (one meter)] with a person who had an unexplained acute respiratory illness that later resulted in severe pneumonia and death.
- Occupation exposure (same as above).

Pathogenesis

Antigenic shift and antigenic drift. Influenza A viruses have a remarkable ability to undergo periodic changes in the antigenic characteristics of the HA and NA envelope glycoproteins. Major changes in these glycoproteins are referred to as antigenic shifts while minor changes are called antigenic drift. Antigenic shifts are associated with epidemics and pandemics of influenza A; for example, the extremely severe and extensive Spanish influenza pandemic of 1918 was related to viral changes in both the HA and the NA glycoproteins. In contrast, antigenic drifts viral changes that result in more localized outbreaks.

Virulence factors. Studies of isolated avian influenza A (H5N1), from patients identified in the 1997 outbreak, revealed that the highly cleaved HA was activated by multiple cellular protease and that specific substitution in the polymerase basic protein 2 could enhance its replication. A substitution in the non-structural protein-1 can increase resistance to inhibition by interferons and tumor necrosis factor-α (TNF-α).[11] Furthermore, the virus can induce several types of cytokines resulting in inflammation and possess the polybasic amino acid sequence at the HA cleavage site that is associated with visceral dissemination in avian species, mammals and humans.[11]

Host-immune responses. The innate immune responses to influenza A (H5N1) may contribute to disease pathogenesis. In the 1997 outbreaks, elevated blood level of interleukin-6, TNF-α, interferon-γ, and soluble interleukin-2 receptor were observed in patients acutely ill with H5N1 infection.[11] Inflammatory mediators such as interleukin-6, interleukin-8, interleukin-1β, and monocyte chemoattractant protein-1 were found to be higher among patients who died than among those who survived.[11]

Clinical Presentation

The history and physical examination. The clinical manifestations of H5N1 infection in humans range from asymptomatic infections to mild upper respiratory symptoms, pneumonia, adult respiratory distress syndrome (ARDS) and multisystem organ failure (MOF). The ratio of symptomatic cases to asymptomatic cases is not known because of imprecise denominator data (asymptomatic cases).[3] Mild cases of infection have been more likely to be reported in young children whereas case detection in adults has predominantly been hospital based.[24] Early clinical presentations include fever (typically >38°C), headache, sore throat, cough, rhinitis, malaise, myalgias and watery, non-mucoid, bloody diarrhea (Table 3). Except for the watery diarrhea, these symptoms are similar to those associated with prevailing human influenza virus subtype H1N1 and H3N2 infections.[11] Symptoms such as conjunctivitis, abdominal pain, nausea, vomiting, chest pain, epistaxis and gum bleeding are seen only in some patients. Notably, two atypical cases of H5N1 infection have been reported. The first atypical case was a Thai woman who presented with diarrhea, nausea and vomiting without respiratory tract symptoms.[25] The second case was a child in southern Vietnam who had severe watery diarrhea without apparent respiratory illnesses, followed by seizures and a rapidly progressive coma mimicking acute encephalitis.[23] In severe cases, the patients usually have rapid clinical progression within one week of symptom onset.[3] Symptoms include dyspnea (at a median of five days after illness onset), respiratory distress, bloody or non-bloody sputum production and a progressive pneumonic process with or without superimposed bacterial infection and ARDS (Table 3).[11] Multisystem organ failure with renal dysfunction, cardiac compromise (including cardiac dilatation and supraventricular tachyarrhythmia), has been commonly reported in severe cases.[11] Risk factors associated with severe diseases and poor outcome of H5N1 infection include older age, delayed clinical presentation, pneumonia, leukopenia, lymphopenia and development of ARDS.[24] Complications include ventilator-associated pneumonia, pulmonary hemorrhage, pneumothorax and sepsis syndrome without documented bacteremia.[11]

Laboratory and radiographic data. Common laboratory findings in patients with H5N1 infection are leukopenia, particularly lymphopenia with or

Table 3: Comparison of mild-to-moderate and severe disease from H5N1 infection.

Organ system	Mild-moderate infection	Severe infection
Constitutional	Fever, headache, malaise, myalgia	Fever, headache, malaise, myalgia
Respiratory	Rhinitis, cough, sore throat	Dyspnea, pneumonia, bloody sputum, ARDS
Cardiac	None	Cardiac dilatation, arrhythmia
Gastrointestinal	Abdominal pain, nausea, vomiting, diarrhea	Severe diarrhea
Neurological	None	Seizure, altered mental status

Note: ARDS = Adult respiratory distress syndrome.

without inversion of the CD4:CD8 ratio, mild to moderate thrombocytopenia, mildly elevated transaminases, elevated creatinine, hyperglycemia and negative bacterial blood cultures. In severe cases, but not in mild cases, there is early onset (< two weeks) of lymphopenia, severe pneumonia, impaired hepatic function, prolonged clotting time and renal impairment.

Chest radiographs include interstitial infiltration, patchy lobar infiltration in a variety of patterns (single lobe, multiple lobes, unilateral or bilateral distributions), lobar collapse and air bronchograms. In severe cases, infiltrates progress to diffuse bilateral ground-glass patterns with clinical features of ARDS.

Transmission Dynamics of H5N1

Human influenza is transmitted by inhalation of infectious droplets or droplet nuclei, by direct contact, and perhaps, by indirect (fomite) contact and self-inoculation onto the upper respiratory tract or conjunctival mucosa.[11] Infected droplets may settle on conjunctival, nasopharyngeal, or other respiratory mucosal epithelium. The HA of human influenza A virus can adhere to the alpha-2,6-linked sialic acid receptor which is the predominant type of sialic acid receptor on the surface of human respiratory epithelium. Attachment is followed by endocytosis and fusion of the viral and cell membrane, leading to entry of the virus into the cytoplasm. The H subtypes of avian influenza A virus such as the H5N1, H9N2 or H7N7 subtypes will preferentially attach to the alpha-2,6-linked sialic acid receptor present on the respiratory and alimentary epithelium of birds, the ciliated portion of human respiratory pseudostratified columnar epithelium and conjunctiva. These findings may partly explain why these avian viruses can overcome the species barrier and cause human infections. Moreover, during the late phase of infection, ciliated human respiratory epithelial cells appear permissive to both human and avian virus infection, which may provide opportunity for genetic reassortment of avian and human viruses.[26]

For influenza A (H5N1) infection, there are three possible routes of human infection: bird-to-human, environment-to-human and human-to-human (Table 2). To date, consistent supportive evidence exists only for bird-to-human transmission.

Bird-to-human transmission of H5N1. In the 1997 Hong Kong outbreak, exposure to live poultry within one week of the onset of symptoms was associated with H5N1 infection, whereas travel with, preparation of and ingestion of poultry products was not associated with infection.[3] Poultry workers exposed to ill poultry and bird butchering were asymptomatic, yet seropositive, for the H5N1 virus.[11] These findings were similar to those reported for the 2004 Vietnam outbreak.[5] In Thailand, all of the H5N1 infected patients had close contact with ill or dead chickens during a two-to eight-day period before the onset of symptoms.[6] Together, these observational data suggest that bird-to-human transmission of H5N1 viruses occurred and that direct contact with live, ill or dead poultry is the primary route of transmission.

Environment-to-human transmission of H5N1. Given that the influenza A (H5N1) virus can survive in the environment, it is plausible that other modes of environment-to-human transmission exist. Oral ingestion of contaminated water during swimming and direct intranasal or conjunctival inoculation during exposure to water were reported in two infected Vietnamese children who swam in a canal where infected ducks lived and fed.[23] The contamination of hands from infected fomites with subsequent self-inoculation and the widespread use of untreated poultry feces as fertilizer are other possible modes of transmission.[11]

Human-to-human transmission. Findings from cohort studies from the 1997 Hong Kong outbreak suggest that human-to-human transmission may have occurred via close physical contact with infected patients.[3] In a cohort study, H5N1-exposed healthcare workers were more likely to have antibodies [8/217 (3.7%)] than non-exposed healthcare workers [2/309 (0.7%)].[3]

In Vietnam, there were two affected family clusters during the H5N1 outbreak.[5] Likelihood for human-to-human transmission was unable to be determined.[5] There has been no report of a similar illness among healthcare workers who cared for the infected patients, despite the lack of full droplet and respiratory infection control measures early in the outbreak. In a cross-sectional seroprevalence survey, there was no evidence of horizontal transmission among exposed hospital employees.[27]

In Thailand, probable human-to-human transmission of influenza A (H5N1) has been reported.[9] The mother and aunt of the index patient became infected >16 hours after unprotected care of the index case. There were no exposures to poultry. The H5N1 virus from this family cluster belonged to the prevalent genotype Z and there was no reassortment with human influenza.[9] In another study conducted among healthcare workers after exposure to infected patients, no one exhibited fever or influenza-like illnesses during the two-week, post-exposure period and the serologic tests for antiH5 antibody were all negative despite inadequate use of personal protective equipment.[28]

Summary. Epidemiologic studies suggest that bird-to-human transmission is the primary route for H5N1 infection in humans. Human-to-human transmission of the virus has been reported although these transmission dynamics appeared neither efficient nor sustained. There is no evidence that the virus has ever caused more than one generation of transmission. To date, healthcare workers have been at low occupational risk for acquisition of H5N1 infection even when appropriate infection control measures have not been employed. Nonetheless, continued precautions and monitoring are essential in case the H5N1 virus adapts for human-to-human transmission.

Conclusions

The three influenza A pandemics of the 20th century caused great human and economic devastation. In several Asia-Pacific settings, newly-shifted strains of avian influenza H5N1 virus have emerged, attributable to agricultural practices and close proximity of humans, birds and swine which together facilitated viral reassortment. Widespread concern now exists about the ongoing outbreak of avian H5N1 influenza due to potential emergence of a more virulent virus to which the populations at large are not immune. To date, the virus has become progressively more pathogenic in poultry and has expanded its mammalian host range. Nonetheless, there is no clear evidence that the H5N1 virus has the ability to adapt well for efficient human-to-human transmission. History of close contact to poultry or an endemic area, together with clinical and supportive data, allow for early intervention and management. Although epidemic studies indicate that bird-to-human transmission is the only consistent primary route for H5N1 infection in humans, continued monitoring and vigilant surveillance remain prudent for prevention and control.

References

1. Tumpey TM, Basler CF, Aguilar PV, *et al.* Characterization of the reconstructed 1918 Spanish influenza pandemic virus. *Science* 2005;310:77–80.
2. Hien TT, de Jong M, Farrar J. Avian influenza — a challenge to global health care structures. *N Engl J Med* 2004;351:2363–2365.
3. Chan PK. Outbreak of avian influenza A(H5N1) virus infection in Hong Kong in 1997. *Clin Infect Dis* 2002;34(Suppl 2):S58–64.
4. Koopmans M, Wilbrink B, Conyn M, *et al.* Transmission of H7N7 avian influenza A virus to human beings during a large outbreak in commercial poultry farms in the Netherlands. *Lancet* 2004;363:587–593.
5. Hien TT, Liem NT, Dung NT, *et al.* Avian influenza A (H5N1) in 10 patients in Vietnam. *N Engl J Med* 2004;350:1179–1188.
6. Chotpitayasunondh T, Ungchusak K, Hanshaoworakul W, *et al.* Human disease from influenza A (H5N1), Thailand, 2004. *Emerg Infect Dis* 2005;11:201–209.
7. World Health Organization. *Confirmed Human Cases of Avian Influenza A (H5N1) Reported to WHO.* Accessed from website at http://www.who.int/csr/disease/avian_influenza/country/cases_table_2006_01_25/en/index.html on 26 January 2006.
8. Taubenberger JK, Reid AH, Lourens RM, Wang R, Jin G, Fanning TG. Characterization of the 1918 influenza virus polymerase genes. *Nature* 2005;437:889–893.
9. Ungchusak K, Auewarakul P, Dowell SF, *et al.* Probable person-to-person transmission of avian influenza A (H5N1). *N Engl J Med* 2005;352:333–340.
10. Belshe RB. The origins of pandemic influenza — lessons from the 1918 virus. *N Engl J Med* 2005;353:2209–2211.
11. Beigel JH, Farrar J, Han AM, *et al.* Writing Committee of the World Health Organization (WHO) Consultation on Human Influenza A/H5. Avian influenza A (H5N1) infection in humans. *N Engl J Med* 2005;353:1374–1385.
12. Mermel LA. Pandemic avian influenza. *Lancet Infect Dis* 2005;5:666–667.
13. Stohr K. Avian influenza and pandemics — research needs and opportunities. *N Engl J Med* 2005;352:405–407.
14. Center of Disease Control and Prevention. *Avian Flu Outbreaks in Asia and Europe.* Accesed from website http://www.cdc.gov/flu/avian/outbreaks/asia on 25 December 2005.
15. Center of Disease Control and Prevention. *Avian Flu: The Virus and its spread.* Accessed from website http://www.cdc.gov/flu/avian/virus on 25 December 2005.
16. Keawcharoen J, Oraveerakul K, Kuiken T, *et al.* Avian influenza H5N1 in tigers and leopards. *Emerg Infect Dis* 2004;10:2189–2191.
17. Kuiken T, Rimmelzwaan G, van Riel D, *et al.* Avian H5N1 influenza in cats. *Science* 2004;306:241.
18. Van Borm S, Thomas I, Hanquet G, *et al.* Highly pathogenic H5N1 influenza virus in smuggled Thai eagles, Belgium. *Emerg Infect Dis* 2005;11:702–705.

19. Tiensin T, Chaitaweesub P, Songserm T, *et al*. Highly pathogenic avian influenza H5N1, Thailand, 2004. *Emerg Infect Dis* 2005;11(11):1664–1672.

20. Puthavathana P, Auewarakul P, Charoenying PC, *et al*. Molecular characterization of the complete genome of human influenza H5N1 virus isolates from Thailand. *J Gen Virol* 2005;86:423–433.

21. Center of Disease Control and Prevention. *Avian Flu: Avian Influenza Infection in Humans*. Accessed from website http://www.cdc.gov/flu/avian/geninfo/avian-flu-humans on 25 December 2005.

22. Center of Disease Control and Prevention. *Avian Flu: Outbreaks in North America*. Accessed from website http://www.cdc.gov/flu/avian/outbreaks/us on 25 December 2005.

23. de Jong MD, Bach VC, Phan TQ, *et al*. Fatal avian influenza A (H5N1) in a child presenting with diarrhea followed by coma. *N Engl J Med* 2005;352:686-691.

24. Yuen KY, Chan PK, Peiris M, *et al*. Clinical features and rapid viral diagnosis of human disease associated with avian influenza A H5N1 virus. *Lancet* 1998;351:467–471.

25. Apisarnthanarak A, Kitphati R, Thongphubeth K, *et al*. Atypical avian influenza (H5N1). *Emerg Infect Dis* 2004;10:1321–1324.

26. Yuen KY, Wong SS. Human infection by avian influenza A H5N1. *Hong Kong Med J* 2005;11:189–199.

27. Liem NT, Lim W. World Health Organization International Avian Influenza Investigation Team, Vietnam. Lack of H5N1 avian influenza transmission to hospital employees, Hanoi, 2004. *Emerg Infect Dis* 2005;11:210–215.

28. Apisarnthanarak A, Erb S, Stephenson I, *et al*. Seroprevalence of anti-H5 antibody among Thai health care workers after exposure to Avian influenza (H5N1) in a tertiary care center. *Clin Infect Dis* 2005;40:e16–18.

6

Avian Flu: The Indonesian Experience

Nuning M. K. Masjkuri, I. Nyoman Kandun,
Tri Yunis Miko Wahyono and Hari Santoso

Introduction

Avian Influenza (AI) is a zoonotic disease of birds, first detected in Italy a hundred years ago. The first documented AI cases in humans originated in Hong Kong in 1997 in which 18 people were ill with severe respiratory disease, six of whom died. Five years later the same virus struck again in the same territory with two fatal cases, but this time followed by the emergence of cases from other countries as well. Thailand, Vietnam, Cambodia and Indonesia reported AI cases with a high fatality rate. The first human case in Indonesia was reported on 8 June 2005 and died four days later. His death was preceded by the death of his youngest daughter, and followed by the death of his older daughter, all with similar symptoms.

On 13 July 2005 the word "Flu Burung" (Indonesian word for avian flu) hit the Indonesian mass media, and just overnight became the hottest topic in the country. Flu, an abbreviation for influenza is a household name, used indiscriminately for influenza and common cold. Both have been around for as long as one can remember. But the term is always associated with a mild, self-limiting disease with symptoms of fever, malaise, headache and runny nose, lasting for a few days. Death is rare and happens only in the very young or the very old. Yet this particular flu took its toll on the life of a young man and his two daughters, ages one and nine, respectively.

The fatalities yielded an immediate response from the Directorate General for Disease Control and Environmental Health (DGDC & EH), Ministry of Health (MOH), resulting in an extensive investigation. Differential diagnoses for those cases included plague, hanta pulmonary syndrome, Nipah virus infection, severe acute respiratory syndrome (SARS) and avian influenza (AI). As there was no travel history to AI epidemic areas and no direct contact with poultry, AI became the last diagnosis. Specimens taken from rodents around their home were negative for hanta virus or *Yersinia pestis* (the agent causing plague). Suspicion towards hanta was not unreasonable. The symptoms and signs were very similar to those of hanta and a serologic study done in the early 1990s on rodents and longshoremen from several ports in Indonesia, yielded positive results for hanta virus antibody, although only in a small proportion. Plague was considered because *Yersinia pestis* is prevalent in rodents in Boyolali, Central Java.

Specimens taken from two of the three victims (the youngest victim died before a specimen could be taken) were sent to the National Institute of Health Research and Development Laboratory, Jakarta, the Naval Military Research Unit Det. 2, Jakarta (NAMRU), and the University of Hong Kong laboratory for confirmation. The results showed traces of the AI virus, though the absence of the virus in one of the specimens did cast doubt. Thus only one of the first three cases was confirmed. Blood samples and pharyngeal swabs taken from their family and friends were all negative for AI.

On 20 June 2005 the Government of Indonesia confirmed the existence of H5N1 infection in humans, thus making Indonesia the fifth Asian country to report the existence of AI in humans, after China, Cambodia, Thailand and Vietnam. From then on, cases have been sporadically emerging, and in the span of six months (data on 14 January 2006) almost 200 suspect AI cases were found scattered across ten provinces of Indonesia; 19 (9.5%) of them confirmed by laboratory tests.

On 19 September 2005 the Minister of Health declared the condition as a nationwide unusual event. The term unusual event is used to indicate that the central government will provide funding to control the outbreak.

The Unusual Event of the Human Avian Flu in Indonesia

The World Health Organization (WHO) stated that the current AI outbreak started in the Republic of Korea in December 2003, while poultry population in Indonesia has been rampaged by the disease since October 2003. A new and extremely severe AI virus, the H5N1 strain, has caused the largest and most severe outbreak in poultry that has ever been recorded so far. AI epizootics in the poultry started in the western part of the Java north coast, spreading to the east towards Bali, and then on to the north across the Java Sea to Borneo and the southern tip of Sumatra. Between February 2004 and March 2005 the epidemic receded, but the virus continued its spread to South Celebes, North Sumatra, and Nangroe Aceh Darussalam in the north tip of Sumatra. By November 2005, AI was reported in 26 of 33 provinces in Indonesia. The total loss in poultry is estimated to be around 16 million, 4.7 million due to the disease and the rest eliminated to prevent its further spread.

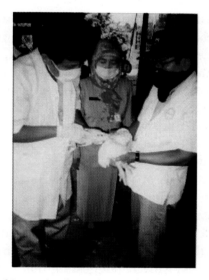

The investigating team taking animal specimens. Source: Ministry of Agriculture (MOA) and Ministry of Health (MOH), Republic of Indonesia.

Even though the victims are mainly chickens, ducks are also healthy carriers of the virus. A study done by Balitbangvet (Research Institute for Veterinary Science) in Bogor, West Java, showed that unvaccinated chicken infected with the AI virus sheds the virus for up to 30 days after infection. Vaccination reduces the shedding period to five days. Virus shedding period for unvaccinated ducks is up to 70 days.

There are a lot of small holding duck farms along the north coast of Java. After harvesting season, some duck farmers used to shepherd their ducks along the paddy fields in the north coast of Java, roaming from west to east. They travel on the harvested paddy fields, allowing their fowls to foray on the remnant paddies scattered in the field, collecting and selling their eggs along the way. When the ducks are no longer productive, they are sold for their meat. Along with other means such as poultry trading between districts, this practice might facilitate the spread of the virus among poultry along the coast of Java. However, this is just conjecture as there is no conclusive evidence so far.

The agent causing AI is a virus from the Orthomyxoviridae family. The disease is prevalent in fowls especially wild birds and water fowls which are the primary reservoirs for the virus. The migration of wild birds and water fowls between islands or continents spreads the disease around the globe.

Indonesia is an archipelago of around 3000 islands in the belt of the equator. Many of the islands are unpopulated and unnamed. There are five big islands, namely Sumatra, Java, Borneo (only the southern part; the northern part belongs to Malaysia and Brunei Darussalam), Celebes, and Papua (only the western part; the eastern part belongs to Papua New Guinea). The country sits right in the path of the migration route of wild birds between China and Australia called the East Asia-Australia Flyway. Some of the small islands such as Rambut islands, several miles off Java's north coast are known as one of the transitory places for migrating birds. They live on the island for as long as two to four months each year. Some of them even breed during their stay.

The virus causing these outbreaks in Indonesia is closely related to the virus strain from Yunnan (China), differing from the one rampaging Vietnam and Thailand. Specimens from the fatal human cases yield a virus closely related in strain to those taken from ducks in Kulon Progo, Yogyakarta (Duck/Kulon Progo/BBVET904) and quails from Cirebon, West Java (Quail/Cirebon/BBVET105), suggesting that virus perpetuation happens within the country, not due to repeated introduction of viruses from migrating wild birds.

The H5N1 virus is found abundantly in the gut of infected birds/fowls, whether ill from the disease or in a carrier state. The virus is shed through saliva and droppings. Thus disease can be transmitted through contact with birds/fowls harboring the virus or through their secretions and droppings. However, transmission from birds to humans remains unexplained.

Conforming to WHO's guidelines, AI cases in humans are classified into three categories, namely suspect AI case, probable case, and confirmed case. Suspect AI cases are those with fever (>38°C), showing one or more of the following symptoms: cough, sore throat, shortness of breath (dyspneu), and at least one of the following histories: contact with confirmed AI case, visiting an affected poultry farm within one week before onset, and working in a laboratory in which the AI virus is handled. Probable cases are those who fulfill criteria for suspects, and one or more of the following conditions: four-fold rise of H5-specific antibody in pair sera, the presence of H5 specific in one serum sample, or disease progresses rapidly into severe pneumonia, acute respiratory distress, or death due to pneumonia of known etiology. Confirmed cases are those fulfilling criteria for suspect or probable case, accompanied by one or more of the following conditions: specimen positive for AI virus, polymerase chain reaction (PCR) positive for H5N1, presence of AI antigen by monoclonal influenza A/H5N1 antibody, or four-fold rise of H5-specific antibody in paired sera.

As of January 2006 there are 19 confirmed AI cases. All of them came from four provinces located in the southwestern part of Indonesia. Provinces contributing AI cases are DKI Jakarta, Banten, Lampung, and West Java. They sit adjacent to one another around the Sunda strait (see spot map). Almost the whole area of those provinces are accessible either by land, sea or air. There is a lot of traffic between them, both for trade and travel. Location and date of onset of the confirmed cases is depicted in Table 1.

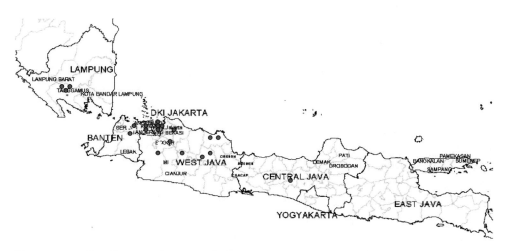

Human case distribution of avian influenza in Indonesia (up to 14 February 2006). Source: Disease Control and Environmental Health (DC & EH), Ministry of Health (MOH), Republic of Indonesia.

Shorter and shorter time intervals between cases reflect the increasing rapidity of transmission. The first case in Banten seemed to be a solitary case (in fact it was a family cluster consisting of a father and his two daughters) indicating the presence of the virus in the area. The second wave started

Table 1: Date of onset and location of confirmed AI cases (up to 14 January 2005).

		Provinces		
Month	Banten	DKI Jakarta	West Java	Lampung
July	2nd	–	–	–
August	–	31st	–	–
September	–	17th	20th, 28th	22nd
October	–	–	19th, 25th	7th
November	–	6th	3rd, 17th	–
December	–	9th, 12th	–	–
January '06	–	8th	7th, 8th	–

in DKI Jakarta and moved to the adjacent provinces. The small number of cases, the scattered location and spread out time interval between cases in each location, suggest no direct link between cases, except those happening within families.

Of the 19 confirmed cases, some appear to be family clusters. The first confirmed cases and his two daughters came from Bekasi (in Banten province), a district adjacent to Jakarta Metropolitan City. They are a family of five, two of whom (the wife and son) were free of the disease and have negative serologic and RT-PCR. The nine-year-old girl was the first to become ill. On 24 June 2005 she had diarrhea and fever, and was taken to a private clinic for consultation. Despite treatment, her temperature rose which was accompanied by cough that prompted the second visit to the clinic. She was eventually admitted to the hospital on 28 June. After two days in the isolation ward, her condition deteriorated so she was moved to the ICU where she died from respiratory distress on 14 July, 20 days after the onset of the disease. Her younger sister became ill with fever and diarrhea on 28 June, she was treated with antibiotics in the outpatient clinic of the hospital where her older sister was treated. When her condition worsened, she was admitted to another hospital and died in the ICU two days later. The father, who started suffering from fever and mild cold on 2 July, was admitted to the hospital four days later and died on 12 July. In this family cluster, exposure to poultry was uncertain. Estimating the incubation period at two to seven days and period of communicability around seven days, person-to-person transmission was possible. However, the fact that the trio was always in close contact with the other two family members who remained healthy and showed no trace of infection suggested that other factors were present to produce successful transmission. This fact is supported by the absence of cases among health personnel working in the hospitals where the AI cases were admitted. One fatal case was a midwife who never had any contact with AI cases.

The other clusters are from Jakarta (a woman and her nephew) and Lampung (a man and his nephew), and two clusters from West Java consisting of one man and his nephew and one girl and her brother. Many clusters consist of an individual with one extended family member, not the most intimate member of the family. The time onset between cluster members varies, from 17 days (cluster from Jakarta), 12 days (cluster from Lampung), six days and one day (clusters from West Java). Again, the data support the peculiar trend of transmission of the disease at the current time.

Information on contact with potential sources of infection is only available for 15 confirmed cases. Sixty percent of the confirmed cases live in areas with a history of infected fowls, 53% had a history of contact with poultry. For 11 (73%) confirmed cases, the specimens taken from birds and ducks around their houses were found to be positive for AI.

The fact that so many farm hands (even those working in the farms rampaged by AI) are healthy while those with minimum exposure became sick has raised so many questions. Risks for contracting fatal disease also remain elusive. The small number of cases with most of them dead, makes it difficult to analyze the difference between survivors and those who died.

Case Management of Human Avian Flu in Indonesia

Case management of AI infection in Indonesia is developed with the assistance of WHO. For ease of decision on management strategy, other than the three categories of cases, another category called "patients under investigation" or "case in observation" is added. This category is intended for suspects waiting for laboratory confirmation. According to this categorization, in the first three cases, the father belongs to the confirmed case category while his two daughters fit into the probable case category.

Hospitalization is imposed for all suspect AI cases, free of charge. Suspected AI cases are admitted to the isolation ward while undergoing additional examination to verify the diagnosis, except those needing intensive care will be admitted directly to the ICU. Patients are put in isolation to prevent airborne transmission which is estimated for up to seven days after the onset, unless fever persists or their condition deteriorates, which will then demand for special care in the ICU.

The current antiviral treatment used is oseltamivir given twice daily for five days. The dosage is calculated according to the body weight. Children whose body weight are less than 15 kg are given 30 mg oseltamivir twice a day; between 15–23 kg, 45 mg twice daily; between 23–40 kg, 60 mg twice daily; and more than 40 kg, 70 mg twice daily. Only 14 out of 19 confirmed cases have information on the antiviral treatment. Of those, 64.3% were given oseltamivir, the rest were either admitted into a local hospital before the antivirus was available or died before getting the drug. Eighty percent of those who did not get oseltamivir died compared to 67% of those who were given the antiviral treatment. The difference is not significant (Table 2).

Antiviral treatment given early in the course of the disease appears to be beneficial. However, starting antiviral treatment in the later phases of the disease does not alter the fatality rate. Unfortunately Tamiflu, the brand name of oseltamivir, is expensive especially for developing countries, and diagnostic confirmation takes up to a week. Delaying the antiviral treatment is hazardous for the patients and prolongs the threat of transmission to those around them. On the other hand, freely administering antiviral drugs to suspect cases who were later found to be suffering from some other disease will strain the already limited health resources.

In addition to antiviral drugs, symptomatic treatment of AI cases is also deemed necessary. Symptomatic treatment includes antipyretics, analgetics, intravenous fluid drip, oxygen, and respirator ext.

All confirmed AI cases exhibited fever of more than 38°C, and almost all were accompanied by cough and shortness of breath. Only a small proportion had sore throat. Laboratory findings showed mostly low counts of leucocyte (leucopenia) and half of them had low counts of lymphocyte (lymphopenia). Chest X-rays showed that the lungs (one or both) were full of infiltrate. Fatal cases were all due to respiratory distress syndrome.

Table 2: Results of oseltamivir treatment on AI patients.

Treatment	Dead	Alive	Total
No oseltamivir	4	1	5
With oseltamivir	6	3	9
Total	10	4	14

Measures to Control the Outbreak in Indonesia

Response to the current situation

Although the case fatality rate was high (12 deaths out of 17 confirmed cases, i.e. 71%), the public reaction was somewhat different from in the case of the severe acute respiratory syndrome (SARS) outbreak.

The first reaction of the public for both outbreaks was similar. Some of the victim's neighbors wore masks, and avoided contact with the family whose member was affected. They also refrained from eating chickens. In an effort to calm the masses, representatives from the Ministry of Health visited some members of the victim's family to show that the risk of human-to-human transmission is low. To demonstrate that fear of chicken meat consumption is unfounded, the Minister ate a meal of chicken in public. Low key reports from the affected neighboring countries also helped in abating the public fear towards AI. The message sent was "No human-to-human transmission is apparent. Although most of the victims died, the number of cases was only a handful. Eating properly cooked chicken will not increase the risk of contracting AI, on the other hand contact with sick fowl will increase the risk."

The message averted panic in the community. But at the same time had the converse effect of minimizing the risks involved and underestimating the potential for a global pandemic, especially among those whose business was related to fowls or its products. Many farmers refused to have their herd eliminated, and some asked for exorbitant compensation for their fowls. In some areas chicken carcasses were thrown into the river, without regard for the safety of their community and environment. Protective clothing was only provided in large and medium farms and most of the time the practice was not imposed. Special efforts had to be taken to stress the threat of the deadly virus for the successful control of the disease.

The Government of Indonesia treats the situation very seriously. On 20 September 2005, the President issued the "President's Instructions" which consist of:

(1) Immediate and prompt measures on infected human and poultry.
(2) Prevent the spread of diseases through localization.
(3) Mobilize funds from each ministry for prevention and cure.
(4) Undertake public awareness campaign.
(5) Establish AI forum for synergizing effects.

The DGDC & EH, MOH, set up an AI Unusual Event Command Post (Posko KLB Flu Burung) immediately. Its office is close to the Director

General's office for accessibility in reporting and receiving direction. It is manned round the clock to respond to any reported AI cases. Information is updated everyday. All reports concerning AI cases are investigated.

The detection time, which refers to the time taken from onset of the disease to reporting to the health office, ranged between less than one day and 13 days. The length of the detection time was partly because of the slow identification of the disease in primary health care. Due to the rapid advancement of the disease, those who were reported more than six days after the onset might already be in the terminal stages of the illness. Administering antiviral treatments at this stage might not be effective.

The rapidity of response, i.e. the period between report and investigation, ranged between zero and five days. More than half of the the cases were investigated on the same day. Specimens were taken not only from the infected individuals, but also from their contacts and surroundings. History of illness and possible exposures in each subject were recorded. However, fear of the neighbor's reaction and the coverage of the mass media which can be disruptive to their daily routines, forced some members of the victim's family to stay in the shadows, thus making it difficult to investigate and prolonged the time lapse between report and investigation.

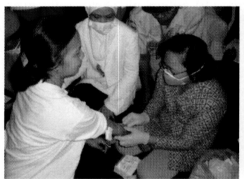 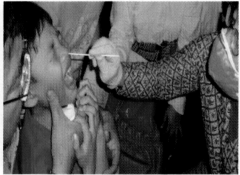

A portrait of the investigation team in the field. The investigating team taking human specimens, i.e. nasal swab and blood (serology) from contacts. Source: Ministry of Agriculture (MOA) and Ministry of Health (MOH), Republic of Indonesia.

Forty-four hospitals scattered throughout 30 provinces in Indonesia previously improved in competency to manage SARS patients in 2002 were converted to referral hospitals for AI cases. Only one referral hospital is designated as the referral hospital for AI cases in each province, except for the following provinces: Riau (six hospitals), DKI Jakarta (two hospitals),

West Java (two hospitals), Central Java (four hospitals), East Java (three hospitals), East Kalimantan (two hospitals), and South Celebes (two hospitals). The number of hospitals in each province reflecting the existence of hospitals with enough facilities and manpower to be able to properly manage AI patients without imposing threat of transmission to their employees as well as to the other patients. The Hospital for Infectious Diseases Sulianti Saroso (Rumah Sakit Penyakit Infeksi Sulianti Saroso or RSPISS) in Jakarta has been designated as the top referral hospital for AI.

The overall health system response consists of the following:

1. Carry out serologic surveys in AI outbreak areas.
2. Distribute antiviral drug (oseltamivir) to all referral hospitals. Oseltamivir is also stockpiled in all provincial health offices.
3. Develop media campaign of AI: Poster, leaflet and guideline book of the most frequently asked questions for community and health personnel. Campaign using mass media are done frequently to rouse public awareness and cooperation.
4. Distribute personal protection equipment. Three thousand protective clothing have been distributed to hospital personnel and investigation team. So far there is no protective clothing provided for individuals handling the infected fowls or involved in the elimination of infected fowls.
5. Holding seminars on AI Surveillance. Several seminars on AI have been conducted for multiple sectors related to health as well as for the community at large.
6. Prepare 100 AI referral hospitals throughout Indonesia and enforce hospitalization of suspected AI human cases free of charge.
7. Stockpile antiviral drug (oseltamivir). The raw ingredient for oseltamivir is found in abundance in Indonesia and the country has secure permission to produce the drug. Hopefully the highly needed antiviral will be available and affordable for all the cases in the near future.
8. Prepare 100 AI referral hospitals throughout Indonesia and enforce hospitalization of individuals suspected of contracting the disease.
9. Strengthen central laboratory at the National Institute of Health Research and Development (NIHRD) as the national reference laboratory for AI by adding necessary equipment (RT-PCR) and material (reagents). In 2006 it will be developed to the status of BSL-level 3.
10. Plan and execute manpower development consisting of:
    a. Study tour of health personnel (port health, laboratory, surveillance and environmental health workers) to Singapore supported by the Singapore government.
    b. Training of laboratory technicians by the NIHRD supported by WHO.

11. Design a pilot project in Tangerang Municipality jointly supported by Singapore and the US, and will be implemented for three years starting from February 2006.

Epidemics due to zoonotic diseases in humans are always preceded by epidemics in the reservoir population, which in the case of AI refers to the poultry population. The most effective measure to prevent such epidemics is containment of the event among fowls through stamping out (total elimination of the fowl population). Stamping out is effective when the outbreak is detected in the early phase and the affected area is limited. Operational costs and compensation for farmers have to be available during these times of emergency. It also needs manpower and self-protection equipment. Stamping out has to be followed by limitation on the poultry traffic to and from the affected areas. These actions pose a heavy financial strain for developing countries. Indonesia like many other developing countries, opted the second best measure, namely selected elimination (depopulation) and vaccination. The widespread affected areas and the wide range of reservoirs make stamping out very costly, not to mention the fact that the efficacy of the result is questionable.

As the AI epizootic in fowls continues, the President of the Republic of Indonesia once again issues instructions to all local officials to participate in control measures. The government also provide funds for the activities including compensation for the farmers. Most government officials agree on the need to relocate poultry farms away from residential areas. However, this is a tall order. In addition, the President has also requested for all veterinarians to be the front line of defense in preventing the spread of AI among fowls.

Prediction and anticipation

There is no certainty in the coming influenza pandemics, but it must be anticipated to mitigate its impact. The uncertainty includes whether Indonesia will be affected by pandemics, and if so, how wide is the affected area going to be? Will it be limited or countrywide? However, the present condition of the country is favorable for the spread of the disease as well as the mutation of the virus. There are small poultry farms and backyard farming in all parts of Indonesia, close proximity of pigs and chicken pens, traditional live markets with goods coming from all over the country, low coverage of vaccination especially in small and backyard farms, etc. Bio-security is almost non-existent. Numerous roads conducive for extensive travel in Java and Sumatra favors the spread of disease.

There are habits in some communities that provide easy transmission of disease to humans, such as consuming seemingly-ill chicken, rare or medium rare meat including chicken, using fresh chicken blood in traditional food, etc. This habit should be banished in order to prevent the transmission of the disease and diminish the chances of the virus mixing with the human influenza virus.

Using an optimistic estimate of 11% attack rate and 50% case fatality rate, the Ministry of Health designed an Influenza Pandemic Contingency Plan with the following.

Strategies:

(1) Maintain preparedness (if Indonesia is not affected).
(2) Determine the size of affected area (if Indonesia is affected).
   Scenario 1: Limited to village level in limited provinces.
   Scenario 2: Limited to sub-district.
   Scenario 3: Limited to district/municipality level in limited provinces.
   Scenario 4: Epidemic of national scale.
(3) Response to:
   Scenario 1: Enforcing village isolation by enforcing Epidemic Law (Law No. 8, 1984).
   Scenario 2: Conducting outbreak investigation and response immediately.
   Scenario 3: Declaring epidemic and enforcing Epidemic Law. The central government mobilizes fund and forces to contain the epidemic and mitigate its impact.
   Scenario 4: Mobilization of national strength and resources including reserved fund and strength (volunteers, etc.) as and when ordered by the President as the Chief Commander during the emergency status of the nation.
(4) Analyze epidemiological situation development and adjust response accordingly.

Policies

A. Prevention and control strategies
   The Government of Indonesia has lined out national strategies to prevent and control AI in humans. Even though the community's health is the responsibility of the Ministry of Health, the government recognized the

importance of cooperation between the Ministry and other related ministries, such as the Ministry of Agriculture and Forestry in controlling zoonotic disease.

(1) Controlling outbreaks and preventing new infections in birds (coordination between Ministry of Health, and Ministries of Agriculture, Forestry and Environment).

(2) Protecting high risk groups with biosecurity (coordination between Ministry of Health and Ministry of Agriculture).

(3) Surveillance (coordination between Ministry of Health and Ministry of Agriculture).

(4) Information, Education and Communication (coordination among Ministry of Health, Ministry of Agriculture, and all related institutions).

(5) Case management and infection control in health care settings (main tasks and functions of Ministry of Health).

(6) Increasing studies and health research. The search for a rapid confirmatory test for accurate detection of AI infection is of top priority. Cheap and effective drugs are also urgently needed.

(7) Declaration of national outbreak of AI.

B. Preparedness strategies

Five key strategies for preparedness and response have been identified to respond to the influenza pandemic and used in our preparedness plan, so that we can treat it as a living document to be continuously revised accordingly:

(1) planning and coordination,

(2) surveillance and early warning,

(3) prevention and control,

(4) health system response, and

(5) risk communication.

Lesson learned

(1) Lessons from SARS have shown that person-to-person epidemics can spread easily and can within a short period infect large areas of the world. An epidemic outbreak in one country is a threat to the whole world. Swift and prompt actions are the most effective and efficient in preventing a global pandemic. Developing countries need assistance in detecting the disease as early as possible (surveillance on the trend of the virus both in poultry and high risk individuals as a sentinel), in

funding (when limiting the spread by stamping out the affected fowls and effective treatment for AI cases), and in future preventive efforts by way of available and affordable vaccines.

(2) There is a need for open communication between countries in order to provide early warning as well as assistance in controlling the outbreak as early as possible before the condition becomes uncontrollable.

(3) The current condition in developing countries provides opportunities to study the disease. For example:

(a) The absence of AI in farmers. Does prolonged contact with the low pathogen virus trigger the development of cross-immunity?

(b) Is there effective alternative medication (traditional) for treatment of AI?

(c) Is there a genetics factors affecting the susceptibility to AI infection?

References

1. Government of Indonesia, Ministry of Health, Centers for Disease Control and Environment Health, AI Unusual Event Command Post (data from field investigations). Unpublished.

2. Akoso BT. *Pemberantasan Avian Influenza pada Unggas. Pandangan dari Dokter Hewan*. Proceeding Seminar Nasional: Prespektif Global Antisipasi Pandemi Flu Burung, Jakarta, 9 December 2005.

3. Patu HI. *Prosedur tetap penanganan Penderita Flu Burung*. Proceeding Seminar Nasional: Prespektif Global Antisipasi Pandemi Flu Burung, Jakarta, 9 December 2005.

4. Adjid RMA, Dharmayanti NLPI. *Pencegahan Penularan Virus Avian Influenza dari Hewan ke Manusia*. Proceeding Seminar Nasional: Prespektif Global Antisipasi Pandemi Flu Burung, Jakarta, 9 December 2005.

5. Mangunnegoro H. *Avian Influenza Viral Pneumonia*. Proceeding Seminar Nasional: Prespektif Global Antisipasi Pandemi Flu Burung, Jakarta, 9 December 2005.

6. http://www.tempointeractif.com/hg/narasi, 16 December 2005.

7. http://www.ppmplp.depkes.go.id/images/m22 s2 i288 b.pdf, 25 September 2005.

8. Peiris M. *Global Pandemic Threat from Avian Influenza H5N1*. Proceeding Seminar Nasional: Prespektif Global Antisipasi Pandemi Flu Burung, Jakarta, 9 December 2005.

9. WHO, SEARO. *Avian Influenza: Responding to the Pandemics Threat*, 2005.

7

Bird Flu in Indonesia

Nugroho Abikusno

Introduction

Bird flu or avian influenza occurrence was first officially recorded in the death of millions of poultry in several areas in Indonesia, especially in the west Java province in August 2003. In January 2004, reported cases of poultry death spread to other provinces in Indonesia such as Bali, west Java, east Java, central Java and west Kalimantan. Initially, the poultry deaths were suspected to be caused by the Newcastle disease virus, however, after further reconfirmation of cases by the Republic of Indonesia (RI) Department of Agriculture, it was verified that the cause of millions of poultry death was the bird flu virus. More than 3.8 million poultry died with the highest number of deaths recorded in west Java — namely more than 1.5 million birds. The government further verified the subtype of the bird flu virus as the H5N1, a contagious subtype bird virus, but not contagious among the human population. To limit the spread of the bird flu virus, the central government prevented its spread by importing bird flu vaccines mostly produced in Thailand. Further, the animal husbandry service conducted mass vaccination of the poultry population in affected areas to prevent further spread of the virus.

The high incidence of bird flu cases among the poultry population in Indonesia is closely related to the animal husbandry system practiced by traditional poultry breeders that is not in compliance with the rules and regulations of the animal husbandry service as well as the non-existence of biosecurity system in poultry breeding farms. These traditional poultry

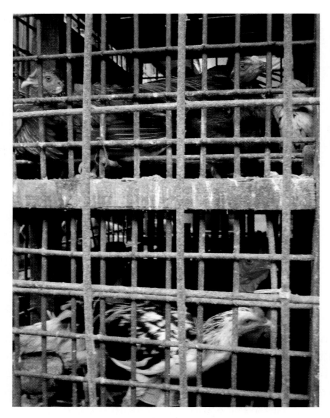

Bird/chicken cages used by traditional poultry breeders. Good sanitation of chicken cages must be maintained. (*Photo courtesy of Dr. Aryo Suseno of the Tropical Disease Division, TCHC Trisakti University.*)

breeders conduct poultry production in a traditional way without regard to modern poultry breeding science and technology. These are the main reasons why many incidences of bird flu are rampant in the traditional poultry breeding community that mostly causes the high incidence of bird flu within the poultry population. These traditional poultry breeders do not thoroughly comply with breeding cage sanitation, routine poultry flock vaccination, and implementation of biosecurity system that could prevent the spread of bird flu among the poultry population.

Bird flu cases were again reported in 2004. Data from the RI Department of Agriculture stated that in 2004, five million poultry exposed to avian influenza were destroyed. The central government through provincial and district governments continued the prevention and biosecurity programs by poultry mass vaccination in exposed areas of Java, Kalimantan, Bali and Nusa Tenggara.

The first incidence of bird flu exposure in humans was reported in south Sulawesi. A man was infected by the bird flu in a poultry farm. Direct contact occurred between poultry to human. The incident occurred in Soppeng district, south Sulawesi that caused thousands of poultry in the farm to be destroyed by burning in February 2005.[1] This incident of bird flu was confirmed by blood analysis in the World Health Organization (WHO) reference laboratory in Hong Kong. However, the farmer had sufficient immunity so that he survived and continued his trade in another district (Sinjai) of south Sulawesi. In the next incident, a confirmed first human fatality occurred in July 2005 and has continued until now.

Cause, Death and Disease Spread

The RI Department of Health is presently reporting the incidence of confirmed cases of bird flu to WHO. The box below contains excerpts of these reports in the form of updates 25–50 between 12 July and 15 December 2005.[2]

- The RI Department of Health reported the first case fatality of Avian Influenza (AI) in Tangerang, Banten province (formerly known as the west part of west Java province) on 12 July 2005. The 38-year-old father was confirmed H5N1 positive and his two daughters had severe pneumonia compatible with H5N1 infection; the one-year-old daughter died on 9 July and the eight-year-old daughter died on 14 July. The remaining four residents of his household remained healthy and showed no symptoms of AI. The RI Department of Health followed over 300 contacts including healthcare workers, extended family members, school and office relations and neighbors. None of these contacts had shown any symptoms of AI and the source of exposure was undetermined (WHO–update 25).
- The RI Department of Health confirmed the second fatal case of AI in Jakarta on 10 September 2005. The 37-year-old woman was confirmed H5N1 positive. The woman lived in an area exposed to chicken and ducks, however, no recent poultry deaths had been reported in the area (WHO–update 29).
- The RI Department of Health confirmed a case of an eight-year-old H5N1 positive boy hospitalized under observation and treatment (WHO–update 31).
- The RI Department of Health confirmed a fatal case of AI in Jakarta on 26 September 2005. The 27-year-old woman was confirmed H5N1 positive. The woman had direct contact with diseased and dead chickens in her household shortly before the onset of the illness (WHO–update 32).

- The RI Department of Health confirmed a case of a 21-year-old H5N1 positive man in Lampung, south Sumatra hospitalized under observation and treatment. The man had direct contact with diseased and dying chickens in his household shortly before the onset of the illness (WHO–update 33).
- The RI Department of Health confirmed two cases of a four-year-old H5N1 positive boy in Lampung, south Sumatra and a 23-year-old man in Bogor, west Java. The first case was hospitalized and recovered. The second case was hospitalized but died on 30 September. Both cases had direct contact with infected poultry (WHO–update 36).
- The RI Department of Health confirmed two cases of a 19-year-old H5N1 positive woman and her eight-year-old brother in Tangerang, Banten province. The first case was hospitalized and died on 28 October 2005, but the second case was hospitalized in good condition. Both cases had direct contact with sick and dying chickens (WHO–update 38).
- The RI Department of Health confirmed two fatal cases of a 16-year-old H5N1 positive girl and a 20-year-old woman, both from Jakarta. Both cases died during hospitalization, namely on 8 and 12 November 2005. Total cases up to this report was 11, and seven were fatal (WHO–update 41).
- The RI Department of Health confirmed a case of a 16-year-old H5N1 positive boy from west Java province. He has been hospitalized under observation and treatment. Field investigation found that chickens in the family household had died before the onset of his illness (WHO–update 44).
- The RI Department of Health confirmed a fatal case of a 25-year-old H5N1 positive woman from Tangerang, Banten province. She was hospitalized and died on 25 November 2005. The field investigation found a history of exposure to sick poultry around her house. Total cases up to this report was 13, and eight were fatal (WHO–update 45).
- The RI Department of Health confirmed a fatal case of a 35-year-old H5N1 positive man from west Jakarta. He was hospitalized on 9 November 2005 and died on 19 November. No evidence of additional cases was detected. The field investigation found a history of exposure to chickens and birds found around his house. Total cases up to this report was 14, and nine were fatal (WHO–update 48).
- The RI Department of Health confirmed two cases; the first case was an eight-year-old H5N1 positive boy from central Jakarta on 8 December 2005, hospitalized on 13 December and died on 15 December. No evidence of additional cases was detected, and samples from pigeons around his household were tested. The second case occurred in a 39-year-old man from east Jakarta on 9 December, hospitalized on 11 December and died on 12 December. No evidence of additional cases was detected. He did not keep poultry in his household, but samples from birds have been taken. Total cases up to this report was 16 and 11 were fatal (WHO–update 50).

Table 1: Summary of confirmed bird flu cases in indonesia 12 July–15 December 2005 based on WHO update reports 25–50.

Case	Gender	Age (yrs)	Location	Status (day/mth)	Contact
1	Male	38	Tangerang	Died (12/07)	Unknown
2	Female	37	Jakarta	Died (10/09)	Direct
3	Male	8	–	Alive	–
4	Female	27	Jakarta	Died (26/09)	Direct
5	Male	21	Lampung	Alive	Direct
6	Male	4	Lampung	Alive	Direct
7	Male	23	Bogor	Died (30/09)	Direct
8	Female	19	Tangerang	Died (28/10)	Direct
9	Male	8	Tangerang	Alive	Direct
10	Female	16	Jakarta	Died (8/11)	–
11	Female	20	Jakarta	Died (12/11)	–
12	Male	16	West Java	Alive	Direct
13	Female	25	Tangerang	Died (25/11)	Direct
14	Male	35	Jakarta	Died (19/11)	Direct
15	Male	8	East Jakarta	Died (15/12)	Direct?
16	Male	39	East Jakarta	Died (12/12)	Direct?

The confirmed bird flu cases in Indonesia between 12 July and 15 December 2005 based on WHO update reports 25–50 are summarized in Table 1.

In the period 12 July to 15 December 2005, there were 16 confirmed cases and of these confirmed cases 68.75% were fatalities. Forty-five percent were males and 55% were females. Seventy-three percent were adults, 18% were adolescents and 9% were children. Twenty-seven percent of fatalities occurred in Tangerang, 64% occurred in Jakarta and 9% occurred in Bogor. The disease began in Tangerang, remained in Tangerang and spread in Jakarta with one isolated case in Bogor. Forty-five percent of fatalities had unknown contact and 55% had direct contact.

In January 2006, another case fatality was reported by the RI Department of Health to WHO. A 29-year-old woman, a midwife working in a maternity ward of a hospital in Jakarta, was hospitalized on 2 January and died on 11 January. Prior to symptom onset, she visited a live-bird market and purchased a freshly slaughtered chicken, however, none of her co-workers showed any clinical signs of influenza.[2]

Pandemic Probability

Based on historical patterns, influenza pandemics are expected to occur.[3] On average, it may occur three to four times in each century when new virus subtypes emerge and are readily transmitted from person to person. In the

20th century, the great influenza pandemic of 1918–19 caused an estimated 40 to 50 million deaths worldwide, followed by pandemics in 1957–58 and 1968–69. Most experts agree that culling of the entire poultry population in Hong Kong in 1997 probably averted a pandemic.[4]

Several measures can help minimize the global public health risks that arise from large outbreaks of highly pathogenic H5N1 subtype avian influenza in birds.[5]

An immediate priority is to halt further spread of epidemics in poultry populations. This strategy works to reduce opportunity for human exposure to the virus.

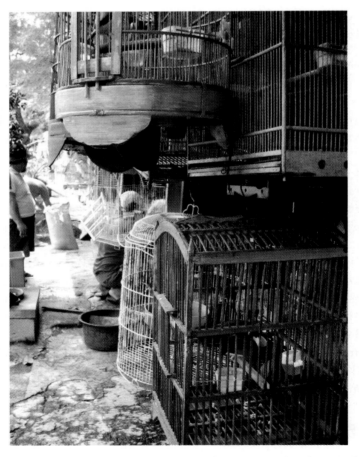

A bird market vending area. Public sanitation must be maintained in these traditional marketplaces. (*Photo courtesy of Dr. Aryo Suseno of the Tropical Disease Division, TCHC Trisakti University.*)

Vaccination of persons at high risk of exposure to infected poultry, using existing vaccines are effective against currently circulating human influenza strains that can reduce the likelihood of co-infection of humans with avian influenza strains.

Workers involved in the culling of poultry flocks must be protected by proper clothing and equipment against infection. These workers should also receive antiviral drugs as prophylactic measure. Two drugs oseltamivir (Tamiflu) and zanamivir (Relenza) in studies have been shown to reduce severity and duration of illness within 48 hours of symptom onset, however, clinical data are limited.[6-8] The main constraints of these drugs are: (1) the limited production capacity and (2) the relatively higher prices especially for developing countries.

Travelers to areas affected by avian influenza in birds are not considered to be at an elevated risk of infection unless directly exposed to infected birds including feathers, faeces and under-cooked poultry meat and egg products. WHO recommends that travelers avoid contact with live animal markets and poultry farms? Large amounts of virus are known to be excreted in the droppings of infected birds. Populations in affected countries are advised to avoid contact with dead migratory birds or wild birds showing signs of illness.

Preventive Measures

Control of bird flu in human population

Direct contact with infected poultry or surfaces and objects contaminated by droppings is considered the main route of human infection. Exposure risk is considered highest during slaughter, defeathering, butchering and preparation of poultry for cooking, however, there is no evidence that properly cooked poultry or poultry products can be a source of infection. A large number of human infections with H5N1 virus have been linked to home slaughter and subsequent handling of diseased or dead birds prior to cooking. These practices present the highest risk of human infection and must be avoided.

The avian influenza H5N1 virus is not transmitted to humans through properly cooked food because it is a heat-sensitive virus. It can easily be killed by heat provided that heat is distributed in all parts of the poultry meat. Thus, normal temperature used for cooking until it reaches 70°C in all parts of chicken will kill the virus.

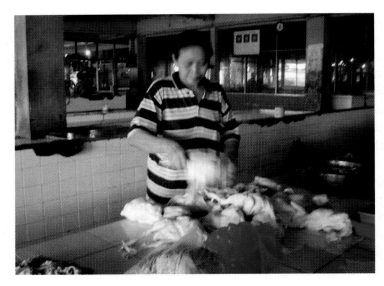

A chicken meat vendor slaughtering chicken for sale in the traditional marketplace. Good personal hygiene and slaughter place sanitation must be maintained. (*Photo courtesy of Dr. Aryo Suseno of the Tropical Disease Division, TCHC Trisakti University*.)

Poultry or poultry products in areas free of this disease can be consumed as usual without the fear of acquiring H5N1 virus infection. WHO recommends that poultry or poultry products should always be prepared following good hygienic practices and that poultry or poultry products should be properly cooked.[9] In general, this recommendation protects consumers from common food borne diseases that may be transmitted through poorly cooked poultry such as salmonellosis.

Most strains of avian influenza virus are found only in the respiratory and gastrointestinal tracts of infected birds, and not meat. However, studies have shown that highly pathogenic viruses including H5N1 have the capacity to spread virtually in all parts of an infected bird including meat. In this case, proper handling of poultry and poultry products during food preparation and proper cooking are most important especially in areas experiencing outbreaks of H5N1 avian influenza in poultry.

Consumers in outbreak areas must be aware of cross-contamination between raw poultry meat and other uncooked foods prior to consumption. Juices from raw poultry or poultry products should never be allowed to mix with raw foods such as vegetables and fruits during food preparation prior to consumption. When handling raw poultry or poultry products, food handlers should always wash their hands thoroughly and clean as well as disinfect food-handling surfaces in contact with poultry products. This procedure should be done directly after food preparation not only of poultry but for all foodstuffs. Always keep your food preparation facilities dry and clean. Soap and hot water will be sufficient for the execution of this task.

In countries with outbreaks, preparation of well-cooked poultry or poultry products should be strictly adhered. The habit of consuming raw or half-raw chicken should be greatly avoided. Consumers must make sure that all parts of poultry and poultry products especially eggs are well cooked. H5N1 virus can survive for at least one month at low temperatures. Common food preservation such as freezing and refrigeration will not substantially reduce its concentration or kill the virus-contaminated meat. In countries with outbreaks, poultry stored under refrigeration or frozen should be handled and prepared with the same precautions as the fresh poultry products. Eggs may contain virus both on the outside (its shell) and inside (white and yolk). Eggs should not be consumed raw or partially cooked. Raw eggs should not be used in uncooked foods.

Control of bird flu in poultry population

There is no drug or vaccine that can treat bird flu infection in the poultry population. Drug therapy and vaccination is mainly directed to prevent the spread of this disease to the surrounding animal and human population. Several strategies that could be implemented in the control of bird flu in the poultry population of poultry farms are:

Biosecurity

The risk is high of bird flu infecting the poultry population. This is due to the relatively long life cycle of poultry (up to 70 weeks) so that it increases the opportunity of being infected by the H5N1 virus. The risk is highest in the productive stage of poultry around 15 to 35 weeks. In this production period, the bird requires more energy for egg production. It is in a stage of low energy reserves resulting in lowered body resistance towards microorganisms. This condition usually affects not only broiler and domestic chicken, but also quail and duck.[1,10] In this case, biosecurity principles should be instituted to prevent the possibility of virus infection. Several biosecurity steps that could be implemented are:

(1) limit poultry or flock trafficking/movement, including its products, feed, droppings, defeathering and cage surfaces;

(2) limit mobility of worker and vehicles within the confines of the farm compound. Unauthorized personnel are not permitted/forbidden in the farm compound. People and vehicles should be disinfected after entering or when leaving the farm compound;

(3) poultry breeders and related personnel entering the farm compound must wear protective clothes and gear such as mask, goggle, gloves and boots;

(4) prevent contact between poultry and wild birds or water birds, mice and other animals;

(5) disinfect all materials, instruments, facilities in farm including poultry cage;

(6) use the disinfectant recommended by the local animal husbandry service such as peracetic acid, hydroxyperoxide, quaternary ammonium preparation, formaldehyde/2%–5% formalin, iodine, phenols and sodium/potassium hypochlorite.

Depopulation

Depopulation is an effort to destroy poultry flock infected by H5N1 virus selectively. The main objective is to prevent disease spread. When a bird shows signs of bird flu infection, such as slime flowing out of the beak or nostrils, or it appears weak, lazy, difficult to feed, and defeathered, then it should be slaughtered and buried or burnt.

Destruction of H5N1 virus-infected poultry flock is by slaughtering all sick and healthy poultry co-existing in one cage or farm. Another method is to dispose affected poultry by burning and burying dead poultry, exposed feed and contaminated instruments. Location of burial site or burning must be within the affected cage area at least 20 meters from the infected cage with a depth of 1.5 meters. If the burial site or burning lies outside this area, it must be situated far from human housing/settlement and its site must have permit and registered by the local animal husbandry service.

Basically, if a case of bird flu occurs in an area and diagnosed clinically, pathologically and epidemiologically as well as laboratory confirmed, then its destruction must be comprehensive, namely destruction of all sick and healthy poultry of the exposed flock as well as all poultry within a radius of one kilometer of the infected farm.

For restocking purposes of new poultry flock, it can only be done one month after decontamination and disposal of the previous infected poultry stock, based on existing rules and regulation issued by the local animal husbandry service.

Vaccination

Vaccination should be done on all healthy poultry in the suspected affected area. Type of vaccine used is killed vaccine officially registered by the government. The vaccination program is directed to: (1) egg producing poultry aged four to seven days, four to seven weeks, 12 weeks, and repeated each three to four months; (2) broiler poultry aged four to seven days; and (3) other birds based on rules and regulations of the local animal husbandry service.

Future Efforts

In the future, efforts to handle the problem of bird flu in Indonesia should focus on managing this disease at two levels, namely the community and individual levels. More emphasis should focus on the individual level for both disease management in the human as well as poultry population.

In the poultry population, surveillance should be focused on identifying the flock of domestic birds (poultry and pets) affected by avian influenza and the possible source of infection, including suspected migratory fowl population if found in the vicinity.[11] The infected flock of birds should be isolated and the confirmed infected flock should be destroyed. In the case of Indonesian traditional poultry breeders, adequate compensation should be given through the animal husbandry services so that the traditional breeders are able to maintain and continue their livelihood in animal husbandry as soon as the bird disease subsides in the poultry population. These traditional poultry breeders should be supervised by local cooperatives facilitated by the animal husbandry service. The advantage of being members in cooperatives for traditional poultry breeders is that poultry production will be standardized based on current poultry production science and technology as well as being members of the cooperative, they will have access to a wider market to sell their produce as well as consumers in the traditional market will be protected from consuming diseased or dead poultry.

Regarding the prevention of disease spread of bird flu in the immediate human population, the tradition of keeping/breeding domestic birds in close proximity to the traditional households should be discouraged because of the dangerous environment it creates and especially to protect vulnerable groups such as small children[12] and women who are particularly susceptible to this disease. Many cases and fatalities have occurred in these vulnerable groups because they are poor, undernourished and living in crowded conditions, where they are living in close proximity to domestic birds and their droppings could easily infect these people through droplet infection.

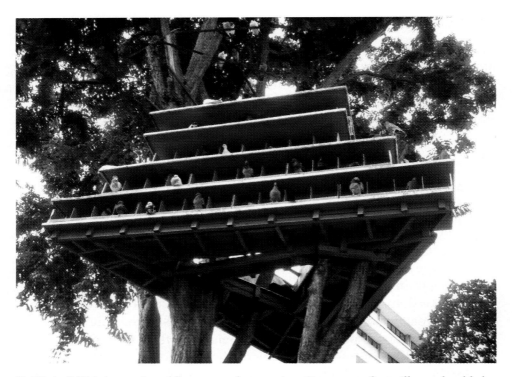

Public (wild) bird cages in public areas such as a university campus. Surveillance should also be done on the migratory wild bird population especially in public areas with a large human population in circulation. (*Photo courtesy of Dr. Aryo Suseno of the Tropical Disease Division, TCHC Trisakti University.*)

At the individual level, the focus is to control the disease in the poultry population through individual traditional poultry breeders, and measures to prevent infection of the individual and his/her community. If a pandemic occurs then it is estimated that 10% of the population could be infected, especially those traditional breeders and their immediate community as well as health and agricultural providers will be the most at risk for disease exposure. Thus, health and animal husbandry education to the traditional breeder community for both individual and family members is imperative that essentially will be focused on poultry health and cage sanitation and food handler hygiene and sanitation both related to bird flu prevention in the poultry and human populations.

References

1. Soejoedono RD, Handharyani E. *Bird Flu*, 2nd ed. Seri Agriwawasan, Jakarta, 2005 (in Indonesian).

2. World Health Organization. *Avian Influenza — Situation in Indonesia (Updates 38–50)*. http://www. who.int/dated 12/10/2005, 1/3/2006, 1/15/2006.

3. Hampson AW. Surveillance for pandemic influenza. *J Infect Dis* 1997; 176(Suppl 1):S8–13.

4. Shortridge KF, Peiris JS, Guan Y. The next influenza pandemic: lessons from Hong Kong. *J Appl Microbiol* 2003;94(Suppl):70S–79S.

5. World Health Organization. *Avian Influenza*. http://www.who.int/dated 12/10/2005.

6. World Health Organization. *Antiviral Drugs: Their Role During a Pandemic* (November 2005). http://www.who.int/dated 1/3/2006.

7. Govorkova EA, Leneva IA, Goloubeva OG, Bush K, Webster RG. Comparison of efficacies of RWJ-270201, zanamivir, and oseltamivir against H5N1, H9N2, and other avian influenza viruses. *Antimicrob Agents Chemother* 2001;45(10): 2723–2732.

8. Ward P, Small I, Smith J, Suter P, Dutkowski R. Oseltamivir (Tamiflu) and its potential for use in the event of an influenza pandemic. *J Antimicrob Chemother* 2005;55(Suppl 1):15–21.

9. World Health Organization. *Food Safety Issues* (November 2005). http://www.who.int/dated 1/3/2006.

10. Kaleta EF. Epidemiology of avian diseases. *Acta Vet Hung* 1997;45(3):267–280.

11. Meslin FX, Stohr K, Heymann D. Public health implications of emerging zoonoses. *Rev Sci Tech* 2000;19(1):310–317.

12. Grose C, Chokephaibulkit K. Avian influenza virus infection of children in Vietnam and Thailand. *Pediatr Infect Dis J* 2004;23(8):793–794.

8

Cultural, Social and Economic Influences of the Flu

Vernon Lee and Kai-Hong Phua

Throughout history, infectious disease pandemics have affected society substantially through direct health effects and from actions taken to try to prevent the spread of the disease. Apart from the obvious health effects, public concern about the spread of a disease results in actions taken by local populations, governments, and international organizations. Most will be targeted at reducing the likelihood of entry of the disease into a country, reducing the spread of the disease upon entry within the country, and reducing the severity and impact of the disease once it has spread. These actions will inevitably result in unintended social and economic ramifications. Social and economic outcomes are highly correlated because changes in each will have profound effects on the other.

This chapter discusses the social and economic impact that pandemic influenza, and more specifically the current avian influenza outbreak, may cause at the global, national, and community level. It will also provide recommendations to reduce the negative impact of an influenza pandemic, and to encourage positive practices that will assist us in combating the disease.

Lessons from the Past

The impact of infectious disease outbreaks can be seen from some historical examples. These outbreaks and pandemics provide a glimpse of the effects that may occur in an influenza pandemic. Although the world has progressed across the centuries, the psychological fear of infectious diseases remains. Actions and policies will be taken across the globe that will result in substantial impact to the local population. We look back at three infectious disease outbreaks and pandemics — the bubonic plagues of the past millennium including the "Black Death" pandemic of the 14th century, the 1918–1919 "Spanish Flu" influenza pandemic, and the 2003 Severe Acute Respiratory Syndrome (SARS) outbreak. These three diseases will show the direct health effects and other effects on society and the economy caused by preventive actions.

Bubonic plagues are a common cause of pandemics in humans. The "Black Death" plague of the 14th century, believed to be caused by the bubonic plague, remains one of the most severe infectious disease pandemics ever recorded. The "Black Death" killed up to one-third of the population of Europe, causing widespread panic across the continent. Bubonic plague was caused by bacteria that were spread by fleas living within rats that were common in populated areas. The disease flourished due to poor hygiene and lack of sanitation. It spread across Europe within five years (a short duration for that era), aided by the major land and sea trade routes that existed across Europe at that time. The pandemic especially affected the poor neighborhoods of cities and other populated areas with crowded living conditions and poor sanitation.[1,2] Due to the lack of understanding of the disease, public health measures instituted were heavily influenced by public perception and fear. Local populations adopted countless measures in an attempt to minimize the effect of the pandemic including the restriction of trade, the movement of populations away from infected areas, and other healthcare interventions. One practice that arose during the pandemic is still in use today. Fear of the disease spreading ashore from ships gave rise to the practice of isolating ships for 40 days away from ports. These ships were only allowed into port when none of the sailors developed symptoms of the disease. The effectiveness of this measure during that time was unknown but the practice, now known as quarantine, has been used ever since. Many of the other public health measures that were used were ineffective because the epidemiology of the disease was poorly understood. Due to the severity of the pandemic and the decline of trade, the economy of Europe was devastated and it took decades for the population and the economy to recover. Resurgence of plague epidemics across Europe occurred until the

17th century, including the great plague epidemic in London in 1665–1666. Although the plague resulting in widespread social and economic damage, ironically it was social and economic development after the industrial revolution that helped reduce plague epidemics through improved sanitation and living conditions.

Another major pandemic that caused global social and economic effects was the 1918–1919 "Spanish Flu" influenza pandemic. It was the worst recorded influenza pandemic in history, and was caused by the H1N1 subtype of the influenza virus. It spread across the globe in less than a year, aided by increased travel and trade during the period. It was estimated to have killed between 20 to 100 million people worldwide, with a case-fatality rate (the probability of death among those who are infected with the disease) of between 2% to 5%. In contrast, yearly influenza epidemics have average case-fatality rates of about 0.05% or less. At that time, the cause of the pandemic was not known and governments attempted to reduce the spread and impact of the pandemic by adopting a variety of public health measures. Many countries and cities imposed restrictions on public activity and encouraged the wearing of masks to reduce the spread of the disease. Some closed public places and schools, and others implemented quarantine measures. Due to the large number of sick which overwhelmed the existing healthcare systems, "influenza camps" were set up in many areas to manage the sick and dying. With the development of science and technology of the 19th century which provided the basis for modern medicine, there was overconfidence on the part of public health personnel regarding the nature of the disease.[3] Many public health measures such as quarantine and the wearing of masks, which may have been effective in reducing the spread of the disease, were not implemented extensively or timely enough to achieve substantial effect. Although the world has changed much since 1918, the "Spanish Flu" pandemic provides us with a model on the health effects that may happen in a severe influenza pandemic.

In contrast, the SARS outbreak in 2003 provides us with an approximation of the social and economic impact that infectious diseases can cause in modern society. Unlike previous pandemics, the SARS outbreak took only a few weeks to cross continents, due to the proliferation of air travel and globalization. Although the outbreak lasted only four months and caused about 8000 cases with 774 deaths worldwide (much less than most pandemics), the social and economic effects were disproportionately larger. The impact of the outbreak centered on the fear of the disease, fuelled by its unknown nature and high case-fatality rates. Many nations distributed travel advisories against travel to affected areas and global travel and trade declined, resulting in economic damage especially to regions affected by the disease. A study by the Asian Development Bank in 2003 estimated the impact of SARS on East Asian economies at more than US$12 billion.[4] Other reports estimate the overall economic cost of SARS at more than US$30 billion.[5,6] Society was not spared either. In Singapore, schools were closed for a few weeks and the public was advised to avoid public congregations. One study in Taiwan found that visits to healthcare facilities decreased by 17% to 35% during the period, presumably caused by a fear of healthcare facilities.[7] This would have prevented the effective delivery of regular healthcare to the population. Similar occurrences may develop during the next influenza pandemic, with similar or greater consequences.

These three infectious disease episodes have provided us with a glimpse of the resultant social and economic effects. With globalization and increased trade and travel across the world, the actual effects will be different from pandemics of the past. The rest of the chapter explores the social and economic impact that may develop from avian influenza and an influenza pandemic.

Economic Costs Resulting from Pandemic Influenza

Infectious diseases affect the economy through direct, indirect, and intangible costs (Figure 1). Direct costs are costs that are attributed to the disease itself or from the measures taken to prevent it. It can be divided into costs for individual medical care and costs to institute public health measures in the community. Costs from individual care can be incurred from outpatient and inpatient medical care including diagnosis and treatment. Medical care also requires utilization of healthcare workers who will have to be protected from influenza, maintenance of healthcare facilities, and administration including transportation to and from healthcare facilities. Some of these costs may be aggregated and included in the hospital bill. Public health measures that are instituted include contact tracing and quarantine, which will require the training of contact tracing teams and also the administration and enforcement of quarantine orders. Research on the new disease will also have to be conducted, as well as health education for the public. During the SARS outbreak, Singapore spent millions setting up the SARS channel and various health education programs through the media. Unique to the avian influenza outbreak, public health measures included the culling of poultry and public education on the avoidance of contact with live poultry. These measures resulted in substantial costs and impacted the lives of those within the poultry industry. The costs arising from the avian influenza outbreak will be discussed below.

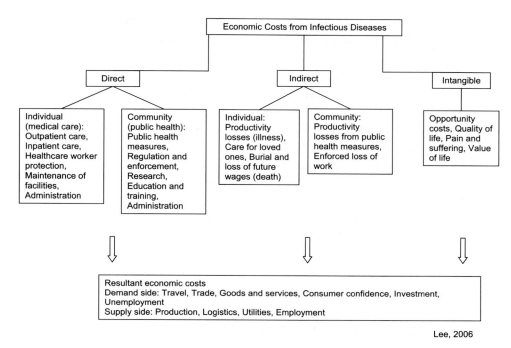

Lee, 2006

Figure 1: Schematic diagram of the cascade of economic costs from infectious disease outbreaks.

In addition to the direct costs from healthcare and public health interventions, infectious diseases also result in substantial indirect costs. Indirect costs are costs that are incurred from the accompanying effects related to the disease or its prevention. At the individual level, productivity losses because of illness are evident and are often greater than the healthcare costs. A study in Singapore estimated that during yearly influenza epidemics, most Singaporeans take on average less than one day of sick leave for influenza illness.[8] However, this will certainly be increased in an influenza pandemic as more severe infections occur and as ill workers are prevented from returning to work for fear of spreading the disease. In addition, symptoms from influenza persist for up to five days, resulting in a reduction in work capacity. As children and the elderly fall ill from influenza, relatives may have to take time off work to care from their loved ones, resulting in further losses in productivity and work days. For patients who perish from the disease, burial costs and the loss of future wages will have to be considered. Loss of future wages are calculated by estimating the lifetime earnings of an individual based on the remaining economic life at the time of death. Public health measures also add to the indirect costs from productivity losses. Contact tracing, for example, may affect work at the affected organization for hours as contacts are identified and separated. In the event of quarantine, costs are incurred through the loss of work. A mitigating factor is that unlike previous pandemics, the Internet provides us with the means to engage in work while physically away from the office. The extent to which this is applicable varies by industry but it provides an option for companies whose employees are ill, quarantined, or remain at home to decrease spread of the disease within the company.

Intangible costs are effects from the disease that are difficult to quantify. Intangible costs arise from the opportunity costs of public health measures, decrease in the quality of life, and the valuation of life itself. Public health measures require substantial time and expertise. These may be used for other purposes if a pandemic did not arise. Unlike commercial entities where opportunity costs are easier to valuate, it is difficult to estimate how much these public health experts may have contributed to society due to the nature of their work. Decreases in individual quality of life are also difficult to estimate because different individuals will assess their loss, pain and suffering due to infection or hospitalization from influenza differently. Costs cannot be placed on such subjective assessments. Similarly, although a person's life can be priced by the future wages he or she generates, the societal value of life cannot be ignored. Using a purely economic assessment of the price of a life, children and young adults will invariably have higher economic value than the elderly. However, the elderly may be prized in different societies for their wealth of experience, previous contributions to society, or simply as part of a complete family. These qualities cannot be priced but must be considered in any policy to prevent the effects of an infectious disease.

All the above actions will cascade through to the overall economy, resulting in demand and supply effects. In severe pandemics, all sectors of the economy will be affected to different extents. Most sectors will be aversely affected but other sectors may benefit from the effects of the pandemic.

The Current H5N1 Avian Influenza Outbreak

The social and economic impact of the current H5N1 avian influenza outbreak has been substantial, especially for the countries directly affected. The direct, indirect and intangible costs from avian influenza are shown in Figure 2.

Direct costs from the outbreak arise from effects of the disease itself and public health measures taken to prevent its spread. Avian influenza results in the loss of poultry and illness among humans. As of 14 January 2006,

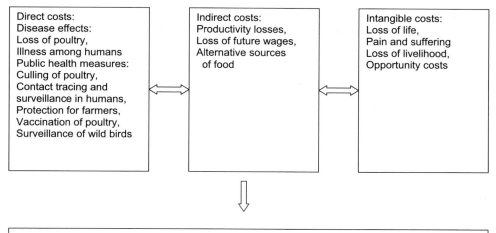

Lee, 2006

Figure 2: Economic effects arising from the current avian influenza outbreak.

there were a total of 148 confirmed human cases and 79 deaths.[9] Almost all of these cases required hospitalization due to severe illness and extensive tests to confirm the infection with the H5N1 influenza subtype. More than 140 million poultry have also died from the disease or have been culled as part of public health measures to prevent its spread.[10] Indonesia alone has confirmed that more than 9.5 million domestic fowl have died since the outbreak in early 2004. Thailand has recently culled 2.7 million ducks to prevent further spread of the disease.[11] Direct economic losses for the entire East Asian region have been estimated at about US$10 to US$15 billion.[12]

Apart from the direct costs, indirect costs arise from productivity losses from farmers being infected by the disease or from public health measures. The culling of poultry, for example, is labor-and time-intensive, requiring the hiring of additional personnel. The culling also destroys the economy of many local villages. The Thai government proposed a US$125 million package in early 2005 to compensate farmers for their losses, and to import frozen poultry to reduce the impact of the destruction of poultry on the local food sources.[11] These costs will increase significantly in the coming years if the outbreak is prolonged. In addition, the effect on certain segments of society, especially on the agricultural industry, could have lingering socio-economic outcomes.

Intangible costs also arise from the loss of life and livelihood for millions of poultry farmers and related industry workers throughout East Asia.

Losing their major source of income is a blow to many locals that cannot be quantified. These farmers may experience difficulty in regaining their lost income in the future.

The fallout of the avian influenza outbreak will affect various sectors of the economy. Those in the poultry trade, including poultry traders or sellers at markets across the region have seen sharp declines in demand and supply for poultry. In areas where there are human cases of avian influenza, demand for poultry has fallen drastically. Associated businesses such as manufacturers of poultry feed will similarly experience a decline in the demand from farmers. Other economic sectors such as travel, tourism, dining, and various financial and investment markets will also be affected by the avian influenza outbreak. Vietnam has already experienced year-on-year decreases in tourism to the country. Businesses in the tourism industry will be hit by the loss of tourists, and dining establishments will be affected by the decrease in the demand and supply of poultry. If the outbreak prolongs or extends, consumer and business confidence may be affected, with further effects on the economy. However, some industries may profit from the outbreak. Manufacturers of influenza vaccines for poultry may experience increased demand for such vaccines from existing poultry farmers. Vietnam has ordered 415 million doses of avian influenza vaccine for poultry to prevent the spread of the disease. It plans to vaccinate all poultry to prevent infection, and is offering a four US cents incentive to farmers for every bird vaccinated.[13] Manufacturers of antiviral drugs and protective equipment are also experiencing sharp rises in orders for these goods.

In the event that the current pandemic spreads, the Asian Development Bank has predicted that a pandemic causing two quarters of economic contraction will reduce the annual growth in gross domestic product in Asia by 2.6%; 2.3% of this will be the result of demand shock (a reduction in demand and consumption of goods and services) and 0.3% will be the result of supply shock (reduction in the supply of goods and services due to decreases in the availability of labor and raw materials).[14] This will cost the region up to US$110 billion. If the pandemic is prolonged with four quarters of economic contraction, economic costs will increase to almost US$300 billion. The economic effect varies greatly depending on the economic make-up of each nation and its reliance on travel and trade. Countries such as Singapore and Hong Kong, whose economies rely heavily on travel and trade, will inevitably feel a greater impact during a pandemic.

The actual cost of the pandemic is also determined by the severity of the pandemic and the resultant economic effects. A study conducted in

Singapore predicted that a pandemic of average severity will result in about 1105 deaths at a cost to the economy of about US$800 million, excluding costs due to public health measures and economic contraction (Figure 1). A severe influenza pandemic with case-fatality rates of 5% (similar to some estimates during the 1918 pandemic) in a population of 4.2 million is estimated to cause more than 60,000 deaths at a cost to the economy of more than US$70 billion.[16] If the costs of public health measures such as quarantine and economic contraction from loss of travel, trade, and investment are included, losses in a severe pandemic may be increased manifold. A similar study by the United States Centers for Disease Control and Prevention (US CDC) found that a pandemic of average severity (similar to the 1968 pandemic) in the US will result in up to 200,000 deaths and costs of up to US$200 billion, excluding costs due to contraction of the economy.[15] The US government has estimated that a pandemic may cost the US economy US$675 billion, including associated economic effects. These estimates show that a future pandemic will result in substantial economic damage, and thus many governments are investing in preparedness plans to reduce the impact of the next pandemic (Table 1).

With the current state of inter-connectivity and complexities among economies, major disruptions to the global economy during a pandemic will likely cause residual effects long after the pandemic has ceased.[19] Global economic contraction, coupled with decreased consumerism and investor confidence during the pandemic may lead to the next global economic depression. Preparation with business continuity plans is essential to limit the damaged caused by the pandemic and its aftermath. This includes minimizing disruption of operations from staff absenteeism, anticipating problems with suppliers, managing decreases in demand, and building safeguards against financial collapse. Governments, businesses, and even individuals should start planning now to avoid panic and economic failure when a pandemic hits.

Table 1: Estimates of the impact of a base-case scenario of pandemic influenza.

Country	Population (million)	Hospitalizations	Deaths	Economic cost (million US$)	Reference
United States	267.6	314,000–734,000	314,000–734,000	71,300–166,500	15
Singapore	4.2	3338	1105	846	16
Israel	6.7	10,334	2855	524	17
Holland	15.6	10,000	4000	–	18

The Influence of Social and Cultural Practices on the Development and Spread of Influenza

Apart from the economic impact, the effects of infectious diseases are also interconnected with the prevailing social and cultural practices. The development and spread of infectious diseases is dependent on the social and cultural activities across the globe and within specific communities.

With the current avian influenza outbreak, most of the cases were individuals who had been in close contact with poultry. The close proximity between humans and poultry is a cultural phenomenon that is especially rampant in rural and even urban communities in Asia. In addition, pigs, a possible mixing vessel for re-assortment of human and avian subtypes of the influenza virus, also live in close proximity to both humans and poultry in many of these communities. This cultural practice may result in the development of the next influenza pandemic. Although much has been done in the areas currently affected by the avian influenza outbreak to reduce the mixing of infected poultry and birds with humans, there are other similar communities where such practices are entrenched in the local populations and will be difficult to abolish. These poultry and pigs provide the main source of food or income for many farmers and developing alternative solutions may be difficult and costly, and may meet with strong resistance.

Apart from contributing to the development of the next pandemic, social and cultural practices also contribute to the spread of influenza. Travel and trade is one of the main culprits in the spread of infectious disease, as seen from the bubonic plague of the 14th century where the importation of the bacteria into Europe and its spread across the continent was aided by trade, following the trade routes of the time. The spread of SARS was aided by the advent of air travel which reduced the duration for spread across continents from years or months to weeks or even days. A study on the spread of influenza across the globe found that with air travel, a pandemic similar to that seen in 1968 will spread across the globe within six months.[20] Even if travel restrictions are instituted during the next pandemic to attempt to retard its spread, the damage to trade and the economy will be substantial and some communities or countries may not subscribe to such drastic measures for a prolonged duration. It will also be difficult to prevent the movement of people around the world, and with many cases of influenza being subclinical or asymptomatic, it will be almost impossible to stop the spread of a pandemic in our current social climate.

In addition to travel and trade, local customs may also aid or retard the spread of influenza within a community. The wearing of masks during a pandemic, for example, may be culturally more acceptable in some communities compared to others. In some polluted cities for example, many commuters already wear masks, including N-95 masks, during their daily activities. These practices may help to slow the spread of influenza and prevent a sudden peak of cases, resulting in a more manageable stream of cases occurring over time. Others may view the wearing of masks during their daily activities as a social barrier and may be less compliant.

Other cultural norms such as greeting practices may also influence the spread of the disease although there are no definite studies on these topics. The shaking of hands, for example, is practiced widely in many cosmopolitan societies. This may aid the spread of influenza through contact with bodily fluids during hand shaking. Socioeconomic factors such as the availability and cost of water and cultural practices will also dictate the frequency of hand washing to help reduce the probability of infection. Other practices such as kissing of cheeks as a form of greeting, common in many Western societies, may increase the likelihood of acquiring disease. On the other hand, greeting practices such as bowing, which is common in Japan, may reduce the chance of spread since physical contact is minimized.

Local dining practices may also contribute to the spread of influenza. Some cultures, such as the Chinese culture, encourage the sharing of food in common servings during meals. In many instances, individuals use their personal cutlery to obtain portions from these common servings, encouraging the transfer of saliva and other bodily fluids. In other cultures, using hands instead of cutlery is the prevailing practice. This is another medium in which virus may be transmitted. Practices such as having individual servings or using common uncontaminated serving cutlery may be more effective in preventing the spread of diseases. These should be recommended as standard dining practices, but may not be well received in many cultures.

Although there are no studies to prove the actual effect on the spread of disease by each of the above practices, these cultural norms will invariably contribute to the way an infectious disease spreads. Alternative best practices will have to be developed and the public must be educated to minimize the spread of diseases in our lives.

Social and Economic Effects of Pandemic Influenza

Social effects that result from a pandemic will likely be substantial, as seen from the SARS outbreak. Social effects that arise are caused by the disease and prevention measures itself, and also from public perception and fear. During the SARS outbreak, there were reports of communities instituting local measures to prevent the entry or spread of the virus. These included barricading villages from outsiders and the vigilante quarantining of individuals who had respiratory symptoms. Such measures, though arguably effective, stem from fear of the disease and may cause more damage than benefits, especially if performed in an uncoordinated and inefficient manner. The SARS virus only infected about 8000 people but the social effects were much more substantial because of the fear that the virus had the potential to result in a pandemic of disastrous proportions. The current avian influenza outbreak has a similar psychological effect because of its potential to result in a severe pandemic, although only a small number of people are currently infected with the virus and there is no known efficient human-to-human transmission.

In the build-up to a pandemic, governments will have to place increased emphasis on public education. Whilst educating the public may be currently conducted in many countries, different social and political cultures will dictate the outcomes. To ensure that the public has access to the appropriate educational tools, and to ensure that compliance to these tools is met, governments and educational institutions must have the mandate and trust of the people. Failure to do so will result in social and economic damages once a pandemic occurs, through public fear, misconceptions, and distrust.

In the initial phases of a pandemic, when only certain countries or areas are affected, travel restrictions will likely be imposed on these areas by other countries. Restrictions in travel, imposed by governments or self-imposed by the people out of fear of infection, will decrease interconnectivity across the globe and cause damage to trade and commerce. Countries that are first affected by the outbreak will bear the brunt of such measures. During the SARS outbreak, Singapore experienced a drop of more than 50% in visitor arrivals within the first month of the outbreak.[21] Vietnam, one of the first few countries to report the emergence of human cases of the H5N1 avian influenza subtype, has already reported decreases in tourist visits over the past year, even though the risk of acquiring avian influenza is minimal.[22] In the event of efficient human-to-human transmission of a novel subtype of influenza, countries may issue travel advisories advising their nationals to avoid traveling to affected countries. Trade and commerce may decrease if countries decide to close their borders to prevent the spread of influenza to their shores. Even though these methods may only be useful during the initial stages of the pandemic, the economic damage they cause can be substantial, especially if the spread of the pandemic is prolonged. As the pandemic continues to sweep across the globe, measures such as travel restrictions and closure of borders will no longer be effective. However, fear and public sentiment may result in the continuation and prolonging of certain measures. Air travel during the SARS outbreak failed to recover quickly in the initial post-SARS period; even though the World Health Organization (WHO) has declared that the outbreak was over. It would be unrealistic to expect that global travel will return to normal during the later phases of a pandemic, even if the chance of acquiring the disease during air travel is no higher than during daily activity. In a prolonged pandemic, global travel may be affected for an extended period, putting the brakes on globalization.

Similarly, businesses will face huge losses from influenza infection and its sequelae, quarantine of staff, and possible decrease in business transactions. The New Zealand government has estimated that at the peak of the pandemic, business may lose up to 40% of the workforce due to illness and to other forms of absenteeism.[23] Businesses should prepare for these possibilities by developing continuity plans which may include dividing the workforce into cohorts, setting up remote workstations including home offices, and educating staff members on the disease and prevention methods. The availability of the Internet will provide businesses with the capability to continue operations to a certain extent from remote locations. This will depend on the nature of the business; for example, financial companies able to utilize the Internet more than manufacturing companies.

On the domestic front, in the early phases of an influenza pandemic, drastic social measures may be taken to attempt to curb its spread. This may include the wearing of masks in public places, prohibition of public gatherings, and the closure of schools. Measures such as the wearing of masks will be accepted differently by different cultures. To many, the discomfort of wearing a mask may be sufficient to provoke flouting of recommendations.

If the SARS outbreak can be used as a prelude to the effects of an influenza pandemic, drastic public health measures will be evident. In the early phases of a pandemic, contact tracing and quarantine measures will be instituted. Although the number of individuals who will be quarantined will be small relative to the general population, media attention on the quarantine will increase the hype surrounding the issue. It is likely in the event of an outbreak that whole areas will be affected. This was seen in the Amoy Gardens residential community in Hong Kong and the Pasir Panjang wholesale market in Singapore. The former outbreak resulted in the evacuation and quarantine of the entire housing community, bringing inconvenience to its population long after the outbreak was over. The latter resulted in the closure of the entire market and the quarantine of many workers, affecting the livelihood of these individuals as well as the public who frequent the market. Each time an area is affected, it may take much longer than the official duration of closure before public confidence is restored.

Similarly, individuals who are infected by the disease, or who work in affected areas, may be shunned for an extended period of time. This is especially possible in the early stages of the pandemic, when most people have yet to be exposed to the disease but have been sensitized by media reports. Such acts will lead to social disruptions and loss of productivity if they occur in the workplace. Unaffected individuals, on the other hand, may avoid public places including taking public transport, and may be absent from work for fear of contracting the disease. This will lead to disruptions to the economy, social interactions and connectivity. These unaffected individuals, fearful of public exposure, may also horde essential items such as food and remain at home. This will contribute to shortages in essential supplies, which will already be affected by reductions in supply and by trade restrictions. Such acts will result in further social and economic damage. To reduce such occurrences and gain the confidence of the population, governments must provide effective public education long before the pandemic occurs. Conducting frequent educational reinforcements before and during a pandemic will help to secure the cooperation of the population.

The closure of schools as a preventive measure will also result in social concerns. Closure of schools may occur when there are pockets of human-to-human transmission within the country, where the risk of a localized outbreak within a school is increased. Closure of schools may also be influenced by public sentiment, including parental fears. Although the closure of schools as a public health measure will decrease in utility as the pandemic spreads across the nation, the re-opening of schools will be a politically sensitive measure. This is especially true since the possibility of outbreaks occurring in schools during a widespread pandemic is as high as any other public gathering. An outbreak occurring in a school will bring unwarranted criticisms against the authorities. The extended closure of schools will result in numerous children being forced to remain at home for a period of time. Continued education of these children will be a top priority. During the SARS outbreak in Singapore, schools were closed for a few weeks and some schools developed their own educational packages to provide continued education for their students during the period. During an influenza pandemic, schools may be closed for extended periods to allay public fears, especially those of worried parents. Even if schools remain open, parents may elect to take their children out of school as a precautionary measure. Providing these children with adequate materials to continue their education during this period will be challenging. In planning for the next pandemic, governments will have to consider developing such capacities to prevent some children from falling behind in their studies. Such material and logistical planning will have to be developed long before a pandemic occurs.

With many children away from school, caregivers will also have to be sought for them. Different cultures and societies will handle this situation differently. In cultures where there are close relationships between relatives, retired grandparents may be the primary caregivers of these children or may be readily available to provide care during a pandemic. However, the elderly are also at the highest risk of developing complications from influenza. In some cities such as Hong Kong and Singapore, live-in domestic helpers may be the primary caregivers during the day. In other situations, parents may have to take extended periods of time off work to care for their children. The resultant loss of work days because of these periods of leave may be greater than the work days lost to influenza infection itself, and must be considered by governments and other organizations.

On a similar note, as the pandemic progresses, large numbers of individuals may be infected with influenza. In most pandemics, the young and the elderly are at higher risk for developing complications including prolonged illness or pneumonia compared to adults, and may require hospitalization. Working adults may have to take time off work to care for their children, parents, or relatives. This will add to the burden on businesses, organizations, and the economy. Additionally, adults who are ill will not be able to care for their young or elderly, leading to care giving issues. This phenomenon may be more pronounced in areas where the healthcare capacity is overwhelmed by the large number of sick requiring treatment or institutional care. If antiviral drugs are able to shorten the clinical course of the illness and reduce complications, then countries with sufficient antiviral drug stockpiles to provide for those affected by influenza will be able to reduce the burden on their healthcare systems. Countries that have limited supplies of antiviral drugs due to lack of funds may also be the same countries that have less developed healthcare systems. These countries can ill-afford an overload of severe influenza cases. Many of the sick in these countries, even those who would usually require hospitalization, may be cared for at home, leading to further losses to the workforce as caregivers are needed.

Another social effect of an influenza pandemic, especially if linked to avian influenza, is on our food consumption. The current avian influenza outbreak has already caused the culling of numerous poultry and many people across East Asia have excluded poultry from their diet, either from fear of contracting the disease or because of the difficulty in obtaining poultry. This is similar to the Nipah virus outbreak in 1998–99 where there were

257 cases of encephalitis and more than 100 deaths in Malaysia, with one death in Singapore.[24,25] Although the number of cases was far smaller than during the SARS outbreak, fear of further transmission prompted the culling of more than one million pigs in Malaysia alone, coupled with the closure of farms and decrease in the trading of pigs across borders. Personal fear also caused a sharp decrease in the consumption of pork, even though distributors and dining establishments ensured that their pork was imported from countries unaffected by the outbreak, and the fact that transmission was through close contact with infected pigs. This will affect some cultures more than others, since different cultures emphasize on different food in their diet. If the current avian influenza outbreak persists and fear is perpetuated by media reports, the exclusion of poultry from the diet can be expected to increase further.

The Influence of the Media

The media has one of the strongest influences on the public and the social actions, due to the ready access by the public to all forms of media, especially the Internet. During the SARS outbreak in Singapore, the government and the media corporations spent millions of dollars on the SARS channel and other public messages and education through all forms of media. This had a strong effect on educating the public on the disease and its prevention, the new healthcare services available, the new laws and advisories, and in providing updates on the worldwide situation and the situation in the community. The media has an important role to play in providing information and updates to the public on developments through the stages of preparation and during the pandemic itself.

However, media publicity can also result in negative social reactions. The Pasir Panjang wholesale market incident in Singapore during the SARS outbreak was emphasized by the media, resulting in heightened awareness by the public. While one of the intents of increasing public awareness was to aid in contact tracing and to reduce the spread of the disease, it resulted in fear and visits to the market decreased even after the end of the outbreak. In the build-up to the next influenza pandemic, there are already numerous reports in the media emphasizing the possible severity. Many articles have compared it to the 1918 "Spanish Flu" pandemic, which adds to the concern. Publicizing the possible severity of the next pandemic has two main outcomes — it encourages people to develop preparedness plans to avert a disaster or soften the impact, but at the same time it creates fear which may result in negative reactions. These negative reactions may include individual hoarding of antiviral drugs or masks, which increases the problem of shortfalls in supply. Sensationalized media reports and rumors during a pandemic, especially on the Internet, may result in people avoiding work, confining themselves at home, and hoarding essential items. This will cause substantial economic and social damage if the next pandemic was similar to the 1957 or 1968 pandemics, which were of average severity and may not warrant such drastic measures to be taken. Sufficient knowledge must be promulgated to the public before rumors take root. The media has a responsibility to provide accurate information to the public prior to a pandemic and to build up the public's confidence and knowledge during a pandemic through education and factual reporting. During the next pandemic, the media can play an important role in minimizing the impact of the disease.

Policy Implications

Government policies will also dictate the impact of the next pandemic, as much as the next pandemic will influence local politics. The SARS outbreak showed that good government policies will lead to success in the fight against the disease. Many of these policies, although effective, will be costly. The Singapore government spent more than S$300 million (US$183.8 million) alone on public health measures during the SARS outbreak to combat the disease. Costs for such measures during the next influenza pandemic should exceed this amount due to the extent and duration of an influenza pandemic. In addition, the government unveiled more than S$230 million (US$140.9 million) in relief packages to soften the impact of the SARS outbreak to individuals and businesses. The assistance provided to individuals and businesses most affected by the outbreak increased market confidence and may have contributed to the support for the government during and after the outbreak.

On the other hand, policies that result in poor outcomes may bring the government involved into disrepute. During the SARS pandemic when the world was caught unawares by a novel virus, the outcomes of many policies were determined not only by astute decision making, but also by chance. Politicians and civil servants have lost their jobs even though they may have acted in the best interest of their community or country, given the limited knowledge available. The next influenza pandemic differs from SARS because its occurrence in the future is a certainty, even though the actual date is unknown. Policy makers have to start developing preparedness plans that will lessen the impact of the next pandemic. Many of the effective tools in detecting the onset, preventing the spread, and containing the effect of a pandemic cannot be built when the pandemic starts. Surveillance mechanisms must be developed and continuously maintained, stocks of antiviral drugs and research into new drugs and vaccines will have to be built, and plans must be rehearsed to ensure familiarity during a pandemic.

Planning for the next influenza pandemic requires commitment over the long term. Due to the threat from infectious diseases, both natural or from bioterrorism, social and cultural norms have to be permanently changed. Preparation for an influenza pandemic, such as building surveillance networks and research facilities, will also be useful against other emerging infectious diseases such as SARS. The trap that policy makers must avoid is the over-emphasis of a pandemic occurring in the near future. Media and policy reports on an impending pandemic may encourage fear and panic. This will result in reactive preparation and abrupt social and policy changes that may not be sustained over the long term. Policy makers should realize that a pandemic may occur this year or more than 20 years later. Policies and social changes should be sustainable over this period and longer to protect not only against influenza but other infectious diseases. This will require budgeting and investment over the long term and continued emphasis on vigilance and preparedness.

With the increased economic and social development across the globe, it will be socially and economically unacceptable not to take any action in the face of impending pandemics. A similar number of deaths as seen in the 1918 "Spanish Flu" or even the 1957 or 1968 pandemics will be viewed as catastrophic in current times, with the advances in medical technology. The next influenza pandemic will definitely affect society, but we may be able to limit the damage but changing our social and economic practices. This will require the collaboration of countries, governments, organizations, and individuals in providing a united effort in combat a future pandemic.

References

1. *The Bubonic Plague, 2002.* PageWise Inc. Accessed from website http://me.essortment.com/bubonicplague_rvdr.htm on December 2005.
2. Slack P. The black death past and present. *Trans R Soc Trop Med Hyg* 1989; 83(4):461–463.
3. Tognotti E. Scientific triumphalism and learning from facts: bacteriology and the "Spanish flu" challenge of 1918. *Soc Hist Med* 2003;16(1):97–110.
4. Fan EX. *SARS: Economic Impacts and Implications.* ERD Policy Brief No. 15, Asian Development Bank, May 2003.0020.

5. Achonu C, Laporte A, Gardam MA. The financial impact of controlling a respiratory virus outbreak in a teaching hospital: lessons learned from SARS. *Can J Public Health* 2005;96(1):52–54.

6. Across the Globe, A Race to Prepare For SARS Round 2. *The Wall Street Journal* 9 December 2003, Vol. CCXLII No. 113:1

7. Chang HJ, Huang N, Lee CH, Hsu YJ, Hsieh CJ, Chou YJ. The impact of the SARS epidemic on the utilization of medical services: SARS and the fear of SARS. *Am J Public Health* 2004;94(4):562–564.

8. Ng TP, Pwee TH, Niti M, Goh LG. Influenza in Singapore: assessing the burden of illness in the community. *Ann Acad Med Singapore* 2002;31(2):182–188.

9. World Health Organization. *Cumulative Number of Confirmed Human Cases of Avian Influenza A/(H5N1) Reported to WHO* (14 January 2006). Accessed from website http://www.who.int/csr/disease/avian_influenza/country/cases_table_2006_01_14/en/index.html on January 2006.

10. *Avian Influenza, Human — East Asia (102): Vietnam*, ProMed Mail, 19 July 2005. Accessed from website http://www.promedmail.org/pls/promed/f?p=2400:1202:9571052644304747848::NO::F2400_P1202_CHECK_DISPLAY, F2400_P1202_PUB_MAIL_ID:X,29747 on December 2005.

11. *Avian Influenza — Eastern Asia (20): Thailand, Vietnam*, ProMed Mail, 12 February 2005. Accessed from website http://www.promedmail.org/pls/promed/f?p=2400:1202:1521639245094448177::NO::F2400_P1202_CHECK_DISPLAY, F2400_P1202_PUB_MAIL_ID:X,28082 on December 2005.

12. European Nations Discuss Measures to Fight Bird Flu. *Vietnam News Agency*, 22 July 2005.

13. Vietnam Confirms 52 Bird Flu Infections. *China View*. Accessed from website www.chinaview.cn on December 2005.

14. Bloom E, de Wit V, Carangal-San Jose MJ. *Potential Economic Impact of an Avian Flu Pandemic on Asia*. ERD Policy Brief No. 42, Asian Development Bank, November 2005.

15. Meltzer MI, Cox NJ, Fukuda K. The economic impact of pandemic influenza in the United States: priorities for intervention. *Emerg Infect Dis* 1999;5(5):659–671.

16. Lee VJ, Phua KH, Chen MI, Chow A, Ma S, Goh KT, Leo YS. Economics of neuraminidase inhibitor stockpiling for pandemic influenza. *Singapore Emerg Infect Dis* 2006;12(1):95–102.

17. Balicer RD, Huerta M, Davidovitch N, Grotto I. Cost-benefit of stockpiling drugs for influenza pandemic. *Emerg Infect Dis* 2005;11(8):1280–1282.

18. van Genugten MLL, Heijnen MA, Jager JC. Pandemic influenza and healthcare demand in the Netherlands: scenario analysis. *Emerg Infect Dis* 2003;9(5):531–538.

19. Sikich GW, Stagl JM. *Are We Missing the Point of Pandemic Planning?*, Continuity Central, 2005. Accessed from website http://www.continuitycentral.com/ArewemissingthepointofPandemicPlanning.pdf on December 2005.

20. Grais RF, Ellis JH, Glass GE. Assessing the impact of airline travel on the geographic spread of pandemic influenza. *Eur J Epidemiol* 2003;18(11):1065–1072.

21. *Economic Impact of SARS.* Joint Media Release from the Ministry of Finance and the Ministry of Trade and Industry, 17 April 2003. Accessed from website http://www.channelnewsasia.com/sars/030417_mof.htm on December 2005.

22. *Vietnam Still a Safe Tourist Destination: Ministries.* Accessed from website http://www.hoteltravelvietnam.com/webplus/viewer.asp?pgid=3&aid=672 on December 2005.

23. *Influenza Pandemic Planning,* Business Continuity Guide. Ministry of Economic Development, New Zealand, October 2005.

24. Update: outbreak of Nipah virus — Malaysia and Singapore, 1999. *MMWR Morb Mortal Wkly Rep* 1999;48(16):335–337.

25. Chapter 1: The emergence of Nipah virus, in *Manual on the Diagnosis of Nipah Virus Infection in Animals.* Food and Agriculture Organization of the United Nations Regional Office for Asia and the Pacific, Animal Production and Health Commission for Asia and the Pacific (APHCA), January 2002.

9

The Consequences and Management of an Established Pandemic of Influenza

Dale A. Fisher

One can only speculate over just how the next influenza pandemic will affect life as we know it. Many debate over whether the current avian pandemic agent, H5N1, will mutate or whether the next flu will evolve from a human form. No one however debates the inevitability; just the timing.

It is said that in 1918 the H1N1 influenza virus pandemic killed more people than the war itself. Dr. Victor Vaughn, Acting Surgeon General of the US army arrived at camp Devans near Boston and is quoted:

> *"I saw hundreds of young stalwart men in uniform coming into the wards of the hospital. Every bed was full yet others crowded in. The status wore a bluish cast; a cough brought up the blood-stained sputum. In the morning the dead bodies are stacked about the morgue like cord wood."*

By October, Boston had been forced to cancel parades and sporting events. Churches were closed and stock market activity was reduced to half days. In October, US congress approved one million dollars to assist in recruiting additional physicians and nurses. Death rates in the major cities approached 1000 per day. The crime rate in Chicago fell by 43%. During the month of October, 195,000 Americans died of influenza. Street celebrations marking the end of World War I in November saw most people wearing a face mask.

Throughout the world, 35 million people in total died of that influenza pandemic. The effect in less developed countries is less clear although millions died via the direct effects of influenza creating a shortage of grave diggers and a need for shallow graves. Perhaps a more significant effect was seen in rural areas where the impact on farming resulted in a great exacerbation in hunger.

The following scenario is personal speculation based on the reading of official as well as individual accounts of past flu epidemics, personal experiences during the SARS epidemic and also some imaginative self indulgence!

In the Beginning

An influenza outbreak, and particularly one emanating from poultry will likely develop in a region of high human density where exposure to poultry by the population at large is a part of daily life. It is also more likely to flourish in a setting where public health surveillance is suboptimal, where government accountability is less rigorous and also where there is a vested economic interest in denial of emerging diseases. It should also be considered that such countries have many extraordinary and real problems which weigh more heavily on its agenda than the theoretical threat of disease and the public health surveillance that this requires. As such, one needs to be wary of unfairly criticizing countries managing issues such as vast populations, complex economies, wars, famine, and periodic natural disasters.

There are therefore reasons quite understandable why infectious disease pandemics are more likely to begin in countries such as China, Russia, Indonesia, Vietnam, Cambodia, and the like.

It is likely however that current awareness of the risks and consequences of a global pandemic will see earlier notification than that in past influenza epidemics and also in SARS which really saw some five months pass before the broader world population was informed. This awareness extends from the public, health service providers, government and also the World Health Organization.

While many regions of the world are being fairly closely observed for evolution of a mutant easily transmissable strain of avian flu, there remain many pockets within countries where activity could take place for months before alarms were raised. A precipitating event will probably be required, such as the defining moment in February 2003 with SARS in a Hong Kong hotel where several people were infected prior to traveling to several destinations around the world including Vietnam, Singapore and Toronto.

The defining event in avian flu will also involve export of the disease and this might be an infected human traveler or indeed a flock of migrating birds. Once this sentinel event has taken place and been recognized the race for containment will commence.

Containment: The First Challenge

One could argue that once this particularly well adapted virus is about then we should quickly skip to every possible and extreme public health measure. In reality, this will not happen particularly in parts of the world never exposed to natural disasters, significant infectious disease outbreaks or the reality of other tragedies such as war or terrorist attacks. Countries that suffered under SARS (both through its human toll and its economic impact) such as Singapore and Toronto will have a public which demands swift and extreme measures to counter an infectious disease threat. Perhaps Europe, Australia and the US will be more resistant to measures which appear draconian particularly if there is a significant impact on lifestyle.

Unfortunately, however, this well adapted virus will be highly transmissible between humans even during the incubation period where symptoms are yet to appear. Transmissibility indeed will be quite low in very unwell patients who are more easily recognizable as having influenza. This is quite opposite to the SARS virus. SARS in fact could be easily contained by quarantining of unwell people.

A disease which is life-threatening (possibly up to 40% mortality rate) together with transmissibility during the asymptomatic phase is a formidable foe. Once this agent is "created and let loose," anything other than extreme measures is pointless. Airport screening may be engaged for a period and may be a useful display by officials for the purposes of public perception, however it is likely pointless. Likewise quarantining of flocks of migrating birds cannot work! In theory, quarantining of passengers traveling from an affected area could work but only for a short period or only for particularly selected regions of the world with a small number of visitors.

Essentially once the outbreak has been recognized, the vast majority of the world's populations will need to protect themselves with a variety of basic public health efforts. These requirements will have a profound effect on our lifestyle that will involve mass education and public acceptance or else the consequences could be merciless.

Because of the propensity for the virus to transmit from apparently uninfected people, the first public health measure will be to prevent the formation of crowds.

A World Without Crowds

Predictably, in the event of an outbreak, society will move to protect its children first and foremost. As such, schools and associated children's activities will cease. Education will need to be delivered via remote means. Internet communications will have an enormous role in simulating classroom activities. Most schools and individual households will not be prepared for particularly sophisticated or interactive internet communication but certainly exercises, essay questions and the like can be delivered electronically and likewise returned to the teacher once complete. Many of the needs for primary and secondary school teaching can be done in this way but only for a short period. The longer the duration of the outbreak, the greater the impact of the outbreak on education. Closure of universities may have a lesser impact as such study is often driven by the individual under normal circumstances anyway.

We will all be frightened to let our children have physical interaction with other children. Sporting and other casual social interactions will not occur or will be minimal. Safe havens will be regarded as the home and open spaces. Walking in the streets, playing in parks, traveling in private vehicles (alone) will all be safe, however circumstances involving close proximity to others particularly physical contact starts to introduce risk. Risk will be weighed against benefits, therefore non-essential leisure activities will be eliminated early. Major and minor sporting events and concerts will be cancelled. People will not attend restaurants. Sitting in a crowded church will be risky and this, like education may see a rapid growth in web- or television-based broadcasting.

People will be very reluctant to take public transport and that decision will also be based on the essentiality. This includes buses, trains and aeroplanes. We will find that people who take public transport or enter a supermarket become clad in personal protective equipment, particularly masks and gloves.

It is difficult to know what policy will take place in prisons. In theory, by stopping visitors this could become another relatively safe haven. Alternatively, increased isolation of prisoners will be another means of stopping transmission within such a crowded institution.

Much of public health management of an avian flu outbreak will revolve around allowing for a world without crowds. We will accept and perhaps even encourage a low threshold to absenteeism. The most essential workers will be health providers for obvious reasons. Elective surgery will be cancelled and inpatient management of less than life-threatening conditions would decrease. People will be uncomfortable being in the hospital when they could be home, even though we know most influenza transmission will take place in the community. There will be significant redeployment of hospital personnel.

Hospital Activity

There will only be a small dropout rate for individual hospital staff *fearing* the workplace. The SARS epidemic taught us that most hospital staff understand their role as health providers and the occasional risk this entails. History tells us that the behavior of staff is extraordinary with their ability to adapt and dedicate themselves to such difficult situations and physical demands. It would not be unusual to see a neurosurgeon collecting a blood sample in the emergency department, senior cardiologists and orthopaedic surgeons may assume roles that are normally the domain of the interns. Infectious disease physicians will have a more consultative role and spend much time making "policy on the run." Management of hospitals affected by the outbreak will probably meet daily to assess manpower needs, supplies and oversee information flow, staff education, morale and the like. Rostering will be interesting. Hospital staff will be reluctant to return home if there is risk that they are incubating influenza. A typical roster will involve seven days work, three days quarantine and four days home. This will therefore involve a two-week cycle if the influenza incubation period is as predicted. Accommodation for staff will need to be provided for all but the home period.

Who Are "Essential Workers"?

The answer to this question is related to the duration of the outbreak. Society can do without anyone for a day or two and perhaps for an event lasting more than one year then almost everyone is essential. We would however estimate that any single wave of influenza will last between six and 12 weeks. For this period there will be an extreme reliance on home-based communications. Technicians involved in telephones, computers, electricity and the like will find themselves in higher demand and very needed. Their work would be quite safe, from an infection point of view as it tends to be done by individuals or small groups.

Providers of food will also be essential in this time period although there will be considerable stock piling in homes, and when one goes shopping the tendency will be to buy large quantities to minimize the number of outings. Fresh food products will be more difficult to manage and people will tend towards tins and frozen or packeted foods. Delivery services will become popular and once again the occupation will be safe. This will be an expanding field and see a re-deployment of staff similar to hospitals. Such occupations will take away from less essential services involving exposure to crowds. Many businesses and retail outlets will close during an outbreak over this period. One can go a couple of months without buying clothes, shoes, kitchen utensils, etc.

Multinational corporations may find it simpler to shift work away from affected regions. Especially if there is a high absenteeism level among staff or indeed it is policy to discourage workers from attending — for instance from Asia to a remote and unaffected location in Australia. This would take advantage of strong existing electronic networks. Another similar measure may be to shift activity from the office place to the home. Providing workers with laptops and mobile phones really means that an individual can be anywhere.

How Will Influenza Affect War?

There are altercations taking place across the world. We know from 1918 that the trenches and the barracks were excellent sites for disease transmission. The December 2005 Asian tsunami had a clear impact on warring factions in Aceh and Sri Lanka. Likewise SARS is recognized as perhaps saving the Air Canada airline from financial ruin by uniting everyone against a common foe.

It is therefore a possible paradox that should influenza rise and be seen as a bigger threat than the traditional enemy then conflict resolution could ensue. Leading up to this time, however, the management of overcrowding of young men will be difficult.

The Stock Exchange

There is probably no reason for the stock exchange to be a 40-hour a week marketplace. Certainly during an outbreak, activity will be significantly reduced as people turn toward survival orientated matters rather than those financial. More can become Internet-based and the hours could perhaps be halved. There is little doubt that there would be a major downturn in most shares. Those involving airlines and the leisure industry will suffer particularly as will the retail sector. Gold traditionally is seen as a safe haven. Perhaps some Internet shares and some pharmaceutical companies will benefit from an infectious disease outbreak, but by large it is likely that there will be panic selling and cashing up.

The Social Impact of an Epidemic

Public education will emphasize the discouraging of physical contact including shaking hands and hugging. People will be asked to try and maintain a distance from others — perhaps two meters. Gloves and masks will be strongly encouraged for those not able to avoid physical contact or undertake distancing. Social contact will fall considerably and life will become much more family- and home-based. People will walk rather than catch public transport and take the stairs rather than the elevator. If they do enter the elevator then they will push the button with their elbow! Social interaction will become even more reliant on phones and webcams.

The Role of the Government

Specifically, the government will have to be very flexible in its leadership over a community in fear. Counseling of employers to have flexible policy to allow people to work from home or be absent will be crucial. The government will have a major role in ensuring adequate and sustained power supply and communication networks. More people staying home will mean greater use of televisions, computers, air-conditioners, etc.

Many families will lose their income earners. This may be temporary because of business closure or permanent through death. The ruin of families and businesses is a need which will have to be recognized by the government and society. Even in the interim some type of support for businesses losing income but still having expenses such as rent needs to be considered. Unfortunately, countries earning less and with populations requiring greater assistance, there will be a diversion of resources from traditional benevolent activities.

Aid from the world's wealthiest to the world's poorest countries will necessarily be another victim of an influenza pandemic, and indirectly it is likely that famine relief and African HIV efforts will be among those to be indirectly influenced by a pandemic.

In Conclusion

Naturally this chapter is speculative. The intention is more to be thought provoking with respect to the broader implications of a pandemic. The societal impact of influenza relates to necessary infection control measures in the public domain. Try as one might, infection control breaches will continue. The outbreak will continue until there is either adequate herd immunity and with a significant toll or if time permits then a vaccine may become available to instill artificial immunity. We do know however that the influenza outbreak will have an endpoint.

We are less sure however as to whether the H5N1 avian influenza virus will ever have a starting point as a cause of a human pandemic. The virus has been with us since 1996 and is yet to manifest significant propensity for human-to-human transmission. Furthermore, no previous pandemic has ever been caused by a H5 virus. Many careers have been forged on the back of anticipating the next influenza pandemic. Billions have been spent on the preparations.

When it comes to infectious disease epidemics, we in the business of predicting the medical future need to remember that the next pandemic from an emerging organism will probably come from a completely unexpected quarter. The SARS outbreak and HIV are testimony to our inability to predict and as such any planning needs to build in a philosophy of flexibility and adaptability.

10

The Socioeconomic Effects of an Avian Influenza Pandemic

Gerald C.-H. Koh and David S.-Q. Koh

"It is only a matter of time before an avian flu virus — most likely H5N1 — acquires the ability to be transmitted from human to human, sparking the outbreak of human pandemic influenza. We don't know when this will happen. But we do know that it will happen." (Dr. Lee Jong Wook, Director General of the World Health Organization, November 2005)[1]

The great uncertainty surrounding the anticipated occurrence of an avian flu pandemic makes any forecast of its socioeconomic implications speculative at best and completely inaccurate at worst.

Predictions of socioeconomic repercussions of an avian flu pandemic need to be grounded on our past experience and understanding of the infective properties of the avian flu virus, mankind's past experience with influenza pandemics and the current situation of the avian flu epidemic in Asia. However, assumptions of similar characteristics need not necessarily hold in future influenza outbreaks.

Avian Influenza

The influenza virus has been in existence for centuries and has been infecting both humans and animals all this time. The avian influenza (also called *avian flu* or *bird flu*) is a contagious animal disease that, until recently, mainly infects birds and some animals. Wild waterfowls, especially ducks, are a natural reservoir of influenza viruses, including the bird flu virus. The birds can carry the virus without manifesting symptoms of the disease and spread the virus over great distances while remaining healthy. Domesticated poultry are also susceptible to avian flu and can cause varying symptoms ranging from reduced egg production to rapid death. The severe form of the disease is called "highly pathogenic avian influenza" (sometimes abbreviated as HPAI). This illness is extremely contagious and associated with near 100% mortality rates among domesticated birds.

Strains of influenza virus are classified into subtypes by their protein coat antigens, namely hemaglutin (HA) and neuramidase (NA). Of the 15 HA subtypes known, H1, H2 and H3 are known to have circulated among humans in the past century and hence, enough people have gained immunity to interrupt the transmission of the virus. This is called herd immunity. However, the current avian flu virus which we are concerned about, the H5N1 strain, is probably unfamiliar to humans and hence, there is unlikely to be much herd immunity.

In the past, avian influenza viruses have rarely caused severe disease in humans. However, in Hong Kong during 1997, a highly pathogenic strain of avian influenza of H5N1 subtype crossed from birds to humans in direct contact during an avian influenza outbreak among poultry. The cross-infection was confirmed by molecular studies which showed that the genetic makeup of the virus in humans were identical to those found in poultry. World health officials became on the alert because the H5N1 virus caused severe illness with high mortality among humans: among 18 persons known to be infected, six died. The outbreak ended after authorities slaughtered Hong Kong's entire stock of 1.5 million poultry.

A disease is said to be endemic if it occurs within a limited population or geographical area at all times. An epidemic is a disease outbreak that occurs suddenly in numbers clearly in excess what is normally expected. A pandemic is said to occur if the outbreak becomes widespread throughout a country, regionally or globally. There are thought to be three pre-requisites for a viral pandemic to occur: (1) the infectious strain is a new virus subtype which the population has little or no herd immunity; (2) the virus has the ability to make copies of itself and cause serious illness; and (3) the virus has the ability to be transmitted efficiently from human to human. The H5N1 virus responsible for the 1997 Hong Kong bird flu outbreak satisfied the first two pre-requisites of a pandemic but the virus has not developed the ability to be transmitted easily from human to human yet.

Mankind's Past Experience with Influenza Outbreaks

Since the 1700s, there have been 10 to 13 influenza outbreaks or probable pandemics, of which three have occurred during the 20th century:
the 1918–1919 Spanish flu pandemic, the 1957–1958 Asian flu pandemic
and the 1968–1969 Hong Kong flu pandemic. Of the three pandemics, the
1918–1919 pandemic was the most severe. The 1919 strain of influenza
was unusual because of the high mortality rate among victims between
the ages of 15 and 35 years. Deaths from influenza are usually due to
secondary bacterial infection but a large proportion of deaths during the
1918–1919 pandemic was caused directly by the virus itself. It appears
that the immune system in young persons, which is usually strong, para-
doxically went into over-drive while battling the influenza virus and progressed into an "immunologic storm" that ran wild, killing the victim.
Nevertheless, the very young, old and those with weak immune systems (e.g. AIDS patients) are still at risk of death from an avian flu
pandemic.

The pandemics of 1957 and 1968 were much milder than the 1918 Spanish flu outbreak and there were several reasons for this: the influenza strains
were less virulent, the patterns of mortality were more typical of a usual
seasonal influenza outbreak (i.e. it was concentrated among the very young
and very old) and doctors were able to use antibiotics. Medical technology and public health had progressed since 1918 and in the case of the
1968 outbreak, some immunity had already been derived earlier from the
1957 outbreak. Global surveillance had also improved, which allowed public health authorities to quickly isolate the virus and manufacturers were
able to provide vaccines for the two strains before the pandemics had
resolved.

The SARS Outbreak

The recent Severe Acute Respiratory Syndrome (SARS) virus outbreak in
2003 saw another type of virus called the coronavirus spread widely in a
short time. However, the SARS outbreak is considered to be "minor" when
compared to the 1918 influenza outbreak because less than 800 persons
died from SARS worldwide but 40 to 50 million people died worldwide
in the 1918 influenza pandemic. However, the rapid spread of SARS to Asia,
Australia, Europe and North America during the first two quarters of 2003
provides valuable basis to predict the socioeconomic effects of a flu pandemic during the 21st century. A study by Lee and McKibbin which used a

global macroeconomic model to estimate the impact of the SARS epidemic on Gross Domestic Product (GDP) in 2003, found the greatest decline in GDP was in Hong Kong where output was lowered by 2.6%.[2] They also estimated that China's GDP declined by 1.1% and both Taiwan and Singapore's GDP declined by 0.5%. A major reason why SARS was quickly contained was people with SARS are not contagious before the onset of case-defining symptoms which helped in implementing effective control measures based on case-identification. However, a person with influenza virus is contagious before the onset of case-defining symptoms, which limits the effectiveness of isolation of cases as a control strategy for this illness.

The Avian Flu Situation from 1997 to 2005

Since the 1997 episode in Hong Kong, there have been several outbreaks of avian influenza outbreaks around the world.[3] Mild cases of avian influenza H9N2 in children occurred in Hong Kong in 1999 (two cases) and in mid-December 2003 (one case). However, H9N2 is not highly pathogenic in birds. Alarm mounted again in February 2003, when a nine-year-old boy and his father became sick with H5N1 influenza in Hong Kong after a trip to southern China. The man who was 33 years old died but his son survived. Around the same period, an outbreak of highly pathogenic H7N7 avian influenza, which began in the Netherlands, caused the death of one veterinarian two months later, and mild illness in 83 other humans. Then, in 2004, the H5N1 virus spread among poultry populations in Southeast Asia, with outbreaks of influenza reported in two separate waves. The first wave in January and February, affected Vietnam, Japan, Korea, Thailand, Laos, Cambodia, Indonesia and China. The second wave, which began in July and continued into 2005, included outbreaks in the same countries and Malaysia as well. Late 2005, the virus spread to Russia, Kazakhastan, Turkey and Romania (Figure 1). Between January 2004 and December 2005, there were 141 human cases of H5N1 avian flu that resulted in 57 deaths (Table 1).

Nearly all of the human cases resulted from close contact with infected birds. However, there is evidence of the first case of probable human-to-human transmission of the H5N1 virus in Thailand in October 2004 but no further human-to-human transmission has been recorded since.

Factors Influencing the Development of an Avian Flu Global Pandemic

Genetic Factors

Because no one can predict when, or even whether, the H5N1 virus will acquire the ability to transmit efficiently from human to human, it is still

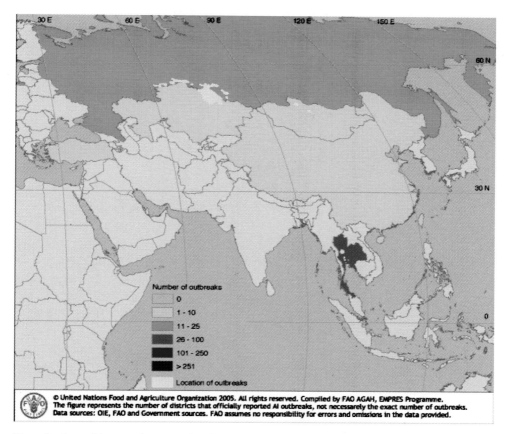

Figure 1: A world map showing the distribution of cumulative H5N1 avian influenza (AI) outbreaks since November 2005 (downloaded on 8 March 2006 from the FAO website http://www.fao.org/ag/againfo/programmes/en/empres/maps.html).

uncertain if an avian influenza pandemic will occur. However, the endemic nature of the avian flu among domestic ducks in rural areas of Asia and the widening presence of the virus increases the possibility of genetic mutations that may make the virus more transmissible. Despite the global concern, some scientists are skeptical of an H5N1 pandemic occurring. Although they agree that a pandemic is a possibility, the researchers argue that the H5 subtype of influenza virus has not shown the ability to pass efficiently among mammals. They reason that since 1997, human and avian influenza strains have circulated concurrently and thousands of workers have been exposed to H5N1 virus during poultry-culling operations in Asia and yet, the H5N1 virus still has not mutated to become efficient in human-to-human transmission.

Table 1: Cumulative number of confirmed human cases of avian influenza A/(H5N1) reported to WHO (downloaded from WHO website on 8 March 2006).

Date of onset	Cambodia		China		Indonesia		Iraq		Thailand		Turkey		Viet Nam		Total	
	Cases	Deaths	Cases	Deaths	Cases	Deaths	Cases	Deaths	Cases	Deaths	Cases	Deaths	Cases	Deaths	Cases	Deaths
2003	0	0	0	0	0	0	0	0	0	0	0	0	3	3	3	3
2004	0	0	0	0	0	0	0	0	17	12	0	0	29	20	46	32
2005	4	4	8	5	17	11	0	0	5	2	0	0	61	19	95	41
2006	0	0	7	4	10	9	2	2	0	0	12	4	0	0	31	19
Total	4	4	15	9	27	20	2	2	22	14	12	4	93	42	175	95

Notes:

1. Total number of cases includes number of deaths.
2. WHO only reports laboratory-confirmed cases.
3. The latest figures are available at website: http://www.who.int/csr/disease/avian_influenza

Early Containment Measures — Is it Feasible?

Two international teams of researchers used computer modeling to simulate what may happen if avian flu were to start being transmitted efficiently between people in Southeast Asia.[4,5] Both their research showed that a carefully selected and orchestrated combination of public health measures could potentially stop the spread of an avian flu pandemic if implemented soon after the first cases appear. Interventional strategies simulated include an international stockpile of three million courses of flu antiviral drugs, treating infected individuals and everyone in their social networks, closure of schools and workplaces, vaccinating (even with a low-efficacy vaccine) half the population before the start of a pandemic and quarantine measures. Targeted antiviral treatment was a crucial component of all combined strategies and public health measures needed to be greatly increased as the virus became more contagious. While the researchers said that implementing such a combination of approaches was challenging as it required a coordinated international response, the models did show that containing an avian flu pandemic at its source was theoretically feasible.

The Pattern of a Possible Avian Flu Pandemic

Although we cannot be certain of the dimensions of a possible avian flu epidemic, past outbreaks suggest the following pattern of events:

1. The virus would spread widely and cross national borders in a very short time.
2. A sharp rise in the number of cases in each affected area would occur within a few weeks with a corresponding increase in demand for medical services.
3. The pandemic would probably spread across geographic areas and vulnerable populations in waves. Each wave could last for three to five months.

The attack rate is the percentage of the population that becomes ill from an infection while case fatality rate refers to the percentage of infected people who die from the infection. Experts generally agree that the attack rates of the past three influenza outbreaks in the last century did not differ markedly and is estimated to be 25% to 30%. Using similar evidence, experts estimate the case fatality rate during the 1918 outbreak to be about 2.5% whereas the case fatality rate during the 1957 and 1968 episodes was below 0.2%.

Factors that suggest that an avian influenza pandemic would be less severe than past pandemics include:

1. Advances in medicine such as antiviral medications which were not available in 1968.
2. Recently enhanced international surveillance systems that have been put in place to trigger an early and rapid response to a new disease.
3. Greater capacity to produce large amounts of vaccines to protect vulnerable populations. However, it should be noted that the months required to produce sufficient quantities of the vaccine would limit its ability to lessen the effects of a pandemic.

On the other hand, there are also factors that suggest than an avian influenza pandemic could be worse than the 1918 pandemic:

1. The world is now more densely populated.
2. A larger proportion of the world is elderly or immuno-compromised as a result of HIV.
3. Faster air travel and interconnections among countries and continents would accelerate the spread of disease.

With so many factors interacting, it is difficult to forecast the severity of an avian flu pandemic with confidence.

The Socioeconomic Cost of Recent Avian Influenza Outbreaks in Asia

The avian flu outbreaks in Asia between 2003 and 2004 resulted in the death or culling of millions of domestic poultry. Direct losses were highest in Vietnam (44 million birds, amounting to approximately 17.5% of the poultry population) and Thailand (29 million birds, amounting to 14.5% of the poultry population). In Vietnam, the cost of the 2003–2004 outbreak was estimated to be up to 1.8% of national GDP which is equivalent to US$450 million.[6] Estimates in Thailand suggested that 1.5% of GDP annual growth was lost. Asian countries like Thailand, Malaysia and Indonesia also experienced financial losses from drop in tourism income.

The impact of the 2003–2004 outbreaks varied along the market chain, and with the type of chain. Large commercial producers specializing in poultry suffered from temporary loss of consumer confidence and preference for other forms of protein. Industrial chains suffered mainly from export loss, including egg traders. However, small commercial and backyard poultry producers lost the least in absolute terms but the most relative to their assets and income. Many had borrowed money to fund poultry production and found themselves in debt when their birds died or were culled. In Vietnam, although a compensation rate of 50% market value was recommended by Department of Agriculture, a rate closer to 30% was paid. Moreover, not all farmers applied for compensation and it took weeks to months for compensation to be issued. For countries like Cambodia which did not have offers of compensation by the government, farmers saw drastic reductions in price of poultry products and quantities sold.

Restrictions on poultry exports from Asian countries affected by avian flu outbreaks in 2004 to mid-2005 contributed to a nearly 20% increase in international poultry prices during this period. On international markets, export shortages due to avian influenza and higher prices led to an unprecedented 8% decline in global poultry trade.

With avian flu becoming endemic in Asia, the poultry sector is expected to restructure in the near future. Consequences of restructuring include fewer backyard and small commercial producers, creation of specified poultry production zones so that production becomes more sanitary and bio-secure, moving of poultry slaughterhouses to outside cities and increasing the number of supermarkets selling processed poultry meat, reductions in free-ranging poultry, more stringent inspections and compulsory strategic poultry vaccination (Figures 2 and 3). These long-term control measures

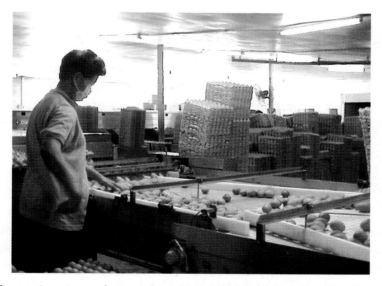

Figure 2: Egg sorting at a poultry egg farm. Restructuring of the industry will result in creation of specified poultry production zones so that production becomes more sanitary and bio-secure.

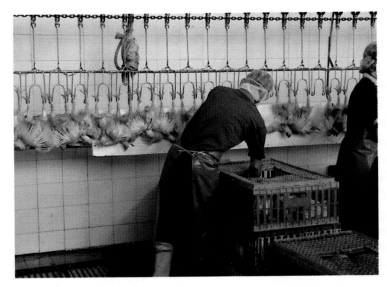

Figure 3: Workers at a poultry slaughterhouse. In addition to improved hygiene measures and personal protection of workers, poultry slaughterhouses may be moved outside cities, while in cities, supermarkets should sell processed poultry meat, instead of live poultry.

could cost countries like Vietnam billions of US dollars, a princely sum that many Asian countries cannot easily afford.

The Socioeconomic Effects of an Avian Flu Pandemic

Little data exists on the socioeconomic effects of flu pandemics and most experts rely on evidence based on the SARS epidemic of 2003.[7] It must be reiterated that it is difficult to predict the severity of a pandemic, let alone its socioeconomic effects. So the ensuing discussion is based on an educated guess.

Short Term Effects

The most immediate impact of a pandemic would be a sudden jump in the demand for medical services. Hospitals and clinics would probably be overwhelmed and surveillance of disease spread and contact tracing would be challenging. Elective surgeries like joint replacements would be delayed and many people will refuse dental work because of risk of contamination. Healthcare workers themselves would be exposed to the disease, resulting in further strains on the healthcare system's capacity: healthcare workers might fall sick, or stay home to care for ill family members or to avoid becoming ill.

People would quarantine themselves and their families by staying at home more. Non-essential activities that require social contact would be curtailed which would lead to significant declines in the retail trade. For example, people would avoid public places such as shopping malls, community centers, places of worship and public transport. Attendance at theaters, sporting events, museums and restaurants would also decline. It is possible that schools might close and even if they did not, parents would tend to keep their children at home. Either event would also result in parents staying home to care for their children even if they were not sick, resulting in workplace absenteeism.

In the current world of just-in-time inventory management of material goods, disruption of supply chains would lead to empty shelves in shops. Stock-piling of basic food, drugs, water, anti-bacterial soaps, face masks, energy and safety supplies would initially lead to shortages and skyrocketing prices. People in panic would shift from animal foods to a more vegetarian diet. Not only would poultry and eggs be shunned, so would other animals which could provide a conduit for disease transmission to humans. Panic-driven behavior may result in constant hand-washing with anti-bacterial agents, discrimination against Asian restaurants or Asians themselves and obsession over media regarding the latest numbers of cases and deaths.

As the pandemic progresses, international travel would dramatically decline, as people avoid avian flu "hotspots" and governments restrict travel, resulting in a plunge in tourism and adversely affect countries dependent on tourism dollars. Businesses would voluntarily quarantine a proportion of their essential staff at dispersed locations to have a stand-by team in case of emergency. People would be unable to make their mortgage and credit payments, and arrears and default rates on consumer and business debt would rise. The general economic slowdown would reduce GDP, dampen business confidence and restrict supply of labor. The stock market would probably fall initially and later rise, as it did in Hong Kong during the SARS outbreak.

The psychological effects of a pandemic will eventually set in. Post-traumatic stress disorder (PTSD) would develop gradually after the first emergencies and could last for an extended period. People will lose confidence and become depressed, tired, irritable, sleep-deprived, over-cautious and paranoid. Traumatized children could suffer from mental and learning problems. Adults would be mourning the loss of loved ones, neighbors and co-workers, and mental problems like depression and anxiety will increase. Certain segments of society, such as healthcare workers and their families, might be shunned by the public for fear of infection. No one will feel safe, a phenomenon that has been kindled in the past by terrorism and war. Personal liberties and freedoms will be restricted as governments impose limitations on movement and civil liberties.

The unemployed, self-employed and uninsured will look to governments for assistance. This will tax the resources of governments at all levels. If an inadequate response to the pandemic occurs, finger-pointing and blame would result in loss of political votes and erosion of political goodwill. Countries may turn against countries and become antagonistic towards international bodies like the United Nations (UN) or the World Health Organization (WHO) for not doing enough to prevent or stop the pandemic.

The poorer countries would be hardest hit, because they have no advanced preparations, effective public health systems and readily available financial resources. For China and India, those who live in close quarters to birds and animals would be especially affected. If the avian flu spreads westwards and affects the European Union (EU), the global market would need to prepare itself for further economic shocks. Such economic shocks include higher meat prices for all other forms of meat in the world markets, lower global meat consumption and a shift in trading patterns to fill the gap left by poultry-producing countries affected by bird flu. Countries which are heavily dependent on EU exports for price stability would see prices for poultry inflate. Many African states belong to this category and sky-rocketing prices will further disadvantage these impoverished nations.

An avian influenza pandemic is considered a shock to the economy and economists classify such shocks as either demand shocks or supply shocks. Demand shocks refer to effects on the economy due to reduction in demand for goods and services due to lowered consumer and investor confidence. Supply shocks refer to economic effects due to decreased numbers of workers staying home during a pandemic and supply of poultry and related livestock. The Asian Development Bank has estimated that a short-lived avian flu pandemic affecting two quarters will result in a demand shock of around US$99.2 billion in GDP for Asia, the equivalent of 2.3% of its GDP. If the outbreak is more severe and lasts for four quarters, the estimated loss would be US$282.7 billion, around 6.5% of Asia's GDP.[8] Socioeconomic costs of an avian influenza pandemic also include direct costs from medical care and public health measures and indirect costs from loss in manpower and industrial productivity (Figure 4).

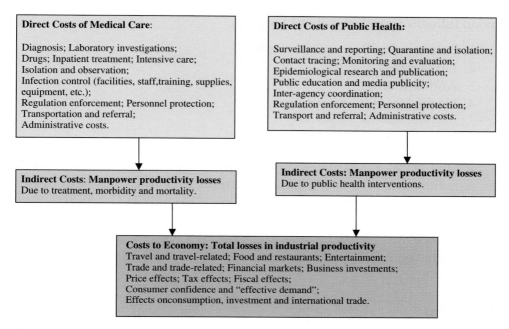

Figure 4: The possible socioeconomic effects of an avian influenza pandemic. Adapted from an eModule on "Lessons Learnt from SARS," National University of Singapore. The socio-economic effects of an avian influenza pandemic can be divided into two levels: healthcare costs (medical and public health) and productivity costs (manpower and industrial losses). Costs can also be divided into three levels: direct costs (e.g. actual expenditure), indirect costs (e.g. loss of productivity) and intangible (e.g. psychological effects).

Long Term Effects

The most important long term effect after a pandemic will be the reduction in the population and labor force. The effect of the reduction would depend on the characteristics of the outbreak. If, for example, mortality was concentrated among the very young and very old, then a pandemic would have a relatively small effect on subsequent GDP growth. However, if the disease struck workers who were in their prime (the "immunologic storm theory"), the effect on GDP growth in the years following the pandemic would then be significant. Orphans from deceased parents would be disadvantaged for the rest of their lives and people surviving the bird flu may suffer from long term effects of the infection (e.g. decreased lung function from scarring).

National Strategies to Contain and Cope with an Avian Flu Pandemic

The Report of the US Congressional Office on the potential avian influenza outbreak recommended that national strategies to contain and manage an avian influenza pandemic should include:[9]

1. Source surveillance and control.
2. Flu vaccines.
3. Antiviral drugs.
4. Healthcare system readiness.

Source Surveillance and Control

When the H5N1 flu virus becomes easily transmissible from human to human, the sooner the fact is known, the more time there will be to gather and deploy available public health resources. Currently, WHO, the UN and other international agencies are trying to contain the H5N1 epidemic among poultry flocks in Asia and have set up monitoring systems to detect new outbreaks (among poultry, among humans and especially human-to-human cases) early.

Flu Vaccines

Currently, there is no licensed human vaccine available for the strain of avian influenza virus now circulating in Southeast Asia. However, there are ongoing efforts to produce vaccines against the H5N1 strain. If a H5N1 flu pandemic occurs in the next few months, producers would probably have to switch their manufacturing from the usual seasonal flu vaccine to vaccines effective against the pandemic strain. Flu vaccine production faces many constraints. Flu vaccines are made from eggs and it is a lengthy process which means the production cannot be scaled up quickly. Moreover, with avian flu affecting poultry and eggs, the egg supply required for vaccine production may itself be disrupted. Intellectual property rights and liability from adverse effects from vaccines are other issues that impede manufacturers from increasing vaccine production.

If policymakers decide that there is time to stockpile vaccines against the H5N1 virus, manufacturers could produce the vaccine during the off season (i.e. the time of the year when they are not producing at full capacity). However, if the pandemic strain turns out to be not of the H5N1 variety, then the stockpiled vaccines would be useless and wasted.

Deciding who to vaccinate is another challenge. Currently, influenza vaccination is recommended to the elderly and those with medical conditions that put them at higher risk for hospitalization and death if they become infected with influenza. However, some critics have argued that younger and healthier individuals should be given priority because they are more mobile than older, less healthy people and are therefore more likely to spread the flu to others. Another factor arguing for giving priority to younger people is that the seasonal flu vaccine produces a weaker immune response in the elderly. Moreover, if the flu pandemic has characteristics of the 1918 pandemic, then the young and healthy are at higher risk of death.

Even if supplies were adequate for all age groups, mass immunization for a potential pandemic still has its risks. In 1976, four US soldiers developed swine flu in an army camp and there was concern that it could become a pandemic like the 1918 Spanish flu. Although some health officials expressed doubts about the likelihood of an epidemic, the government initiated a mass inoculation programme for the entire US population. After hundreds of people receiving the vaccine came down with a rare neurological disease called Guillian-Barre syndrome, the US government terminated the campaign and indemnified manufacturers, ultimately paying US$93 million in claims. Worst of all, the epidemic never occurred.

Antiviral Drugs

Antiviral drugs are thought to be key in the control of an avian flu pandemic. Only two antiviral drugs have shown promise in treating avian influenza: oseltamivir (Tamiflu®) and zanamivir (Relenza®). A treatment of Tamiflu® includes ten pills taken over five days while Relenza® is administered by oral inhalation. The US Food and Drug Administration (FDA) has approved both antiviral drugs for treating influenza but only Tamiflu® has been approved to prevent influenza infection. Because antivirals can be stored without refrigeration and for longer periods than vaccines, developing a stockpile of antivirals has advantages as part of a strategy to control a flu epidemic. However, securing antiviral drugs is not a simple matter of funding because there are currently shortages of them. Moreover, there are limitations to the use of antivirals. Tamiflu® needs to be taken within two days of initial flu symptoms for it to be effective, but many people may not be aware that they have the flu so early.

Some research in animals and recent experience in the use of the drug to treat human cases have also found that Tamiflu may be less effective against the recent strains for the current H5N1 virus than the 1997 strain. Improper compliance to antivirals by some irresponsible individuals during an outbreak may result in the emergence of a drug-resistant strain. Lastly, as experience with Tamiflu® use increases, rising numbers of side-effects are expected to be reported, some of which may be serious.

Intellectual property rights are also an issue with antivirals and some have suggested that governments should confiscate intellectual property rights as a way of accelerating production of antivirals by other companies. However, the long term effects of such a move will make companies less likely to invest in research and development of drugs against pandemics. Another looming concern is that an important active ingredient in Tamiflu® called shikimic acid comes from the star anise, a Chinese cooking herb, of which its supply chain may be disrupted considering that avian flu is most likely to erupt in Asia.

Healthcare System Readiness

Every country's healthcare system would be stretched to the limit in the event of a global pandemic of bird flu. The ability of healthcare facilities to maintain strict infection control measures would be challenged. The sudden surge in health manpower need would be acutely felt among healthcare personnel (especially nurses), epidemiologists and laboratory technicians. Hospitals with an outbreak may be themselves be quarantined and visiting rights of family members of the hospitalized suspended. Communities and healthcare facilities may have to look to other facilities to hold the large numbers of sick and adopt diversion strategies for non-emergency cases. Additional hospital bed capacity may be created by setting up field hospitals and using auxiliary sites such as schools, hotels and community centers. Policymakers may encourage home treatment for those with less serious symptoms to reduce overcrowding in hospitals and to contain the spread of pandemic flu by reducing contact between infected and non-infected individuals. Other social distance measures that may be implemented include closure of public places like schools and other recreational facilities.

Global Strategies to Contain and Cope with an Avian Flu Pandemic

While avian flu is currently concentrated in Asia, wild bird migration is causing spread of bird flu towards the EU (Figure 5).

An avian flu that is easily transmissible between humans would spread rapidly all over the world. The economic cost of an avian pandemic to all countries would be phenomenal and, if allowed to last for months, become exponential. In addition, scientists have demonstrated that an avian flu pandemic can be averted if it is detected early and effective interventions are implemented immediately. A global pandemic will require an international

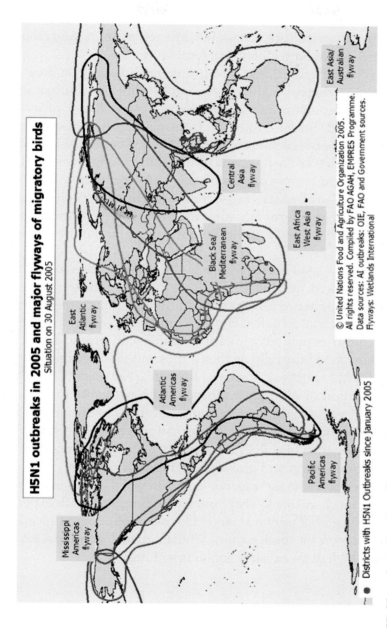

Figure 5: Highly pathogenic avian influenza (HPAI) outbreaks during 2005 and the major flyway of migratory birds. There is a potential risk that HPAI might be carried along migration routes of wild water birds to densely populated areas in the south Asian subcontinent and along migratory flyways to Africa and Europe. Recent outbreaks of HPAI in Russia and Kazakhstan in August 2005 are suggestive of the role of wild birds in the spread of HPAI (downloaded on 8 March 2006 from the FAO website http://www.fao.org/ag/againfo/subjects/en/health/diseases-cards/migrationmap.html).

and coordinated response. Therefore, controlling avian flu is for the global public good and all countries have an interest and obligation to do so.[10,11]

First, the response to the influenza threat would need an integrated cross-sectoral approach, bringing together animal and human health, areas of rural development and agriculture, economics, finance, planning and others. Partnerships are needed at both global and local levels.

Second, there is certainly a priority on curbing the disease "at source" in the agricultural sector, thereby reducing the probability of a human epidemic. International resources are also needed for surveillance of avian influenza outbreaks and human-to-human transmission. It is also important to strike a balance between short and long term measures. Avian flu is becoming endemic in parts of East Asia and will require a long term effort to suppress it. Meanwhile, a human pandemic may still emerge from a different strain of flu virus. Thus it makes sense for the international community to also undertake broad long term measures to strengthen the institutional, regulatory and technical capacity of the animal health, human health and other relevant sectors in Asia.

Third, while country-level preparedness and leadership is essential for success, it must be backed by global resources. Even though the benefits of containing a pandemic are overwhelming, individual governments may still be daunted by the social, political and economic costs of various policy measures. Richer countries may have to support poorer countries in financial and non-financial means in the fight against a flu pandemic, for the sake of global good. The Global Outbreak Alert and Response Network (GOARN), a technical collaboration of existing institutions and networks that pools human and technical resources for the rapid identification, confirmation and response to disease outbreaks, is one such international body that supports global preparedness against bird flu. However, for such an organization to succeed, open communication and global cooperation is essential.

Lastly, there is a critical role for research to fill some of the gaps in knowledge, as well as for mechanisms to share information rapidly with experts, policymakers and the global public at large. Honest public communication will be critical as shown by the lesson of China's denial of a local SARS outbreak initially which delayed early containment measures.

Conclusion

It is difficult to predict whether an avian influenza pandemic will occur, let alone forecast its possible socioeconomic effects. Nevertheless, drawing upon experience with influenza pandemics in the past century and the recent SARS outbreak, a pandemic involving an avian flu virus that is easily transmissible between humans would be catastrophic to world health and economy. However, unlike in the past, we have the prior knowledge of a possible impending pandemic and the knowledge of how to contain and control it. Preparedness, vigilance and cooperation, on a local and global levels, are probably our best weapons against a deadly bird flu pandemic.

Chapter Summary

- Currently, H5N1 avian flu virus is limited to outbreaks among poultry and persons in direct contact to infected poultry.
- However, human-to-human transmission of the virus may result in an Asian and later, global pandemic.
- The severity of such a pandemic is uncertain and hence, prediction of the socioeconomic costs is uncertain.
- Nevertheless, a pandemic will have far-reaching social effects and a high economic cost to Asia and the world.
- National strategies such as source surveillance, flu vaccination, antiviral medications and healthcare system readiness are important.
- International strategies such as early integrated response, curbing the disease outbreak at source, utilization of global resources and continued research are also critical.

References

1. Lee JW. *Opening Remarks at the Meeting on Avian Influenza and Pandemic Human Influenza*. Accessed from website http://www.who.int/dg/lee/speeches/2005/flupandemicgeneva/en/print.html on 9 November 2005.
2. Lee JW, McKibbin W. *Globalisation and Disease: The Case of SARS*. Working Paper No. 2003/16, Australian University Press, 2003.
3. World Health Organization. *Avian Influenza ("Bird Flu") and the Significance of Its Transmission to Humans*, 15 January 2004. Accessed from website http://www.who.int/mediacentre/factsheets/avian_influenza/en/print.html on 30 December 2005.
4. Ferguson NM, Cummings DAT, Cauchemez S, Fraser C, Riley S, Meeyai A, Iamsirithaworn S, Burke DS. Strategies for containing an emerging influenza pandemic in Southeast Asia. *Nature* 2005;437/8:209–214 (doi:10.1013/nature04017).
5. Longini IM, Nizam A, Xu S, Ungchusak K, Hanshaoworakul W, Cummings DAT, Halloran ME. Containing pandemic influenza at the source. *Science* 2005;309:1083–1087.

6. McLeod A, Morgan N, Praksah A, Hinrichs J. *Economic and Social Impacts of Avian Influenza*. Food and Agriculture Office Emergency Centre for Transboundary Animal Diseases Operations (ECTAD), November 2005. Accessed from website http://www.fao.org/ag/againfo/subjects/en/health/diseases-cards/avian_recomm.html on 20 December 2005.

7. Cooper S, Coxe D. *BMO Nesbitt Burns Research: An Investor's Guide to Avian Flu*. Special Report, August 2005. Accessed from website http://crofsblogs.typepad.com/h5n1/2005/08/investors_guide.html on 20 December 2005.

8. Bloom E, de Wit V, Carangal-San Jose MJ. *Economics and Research Department Policy Brief: Potential Economic Impact of an Avian Flu Pandemic on Asia*, November 2005. Accessed from website http://www.asia-studies.com/policybrief.html on 20 December 2005.

9. US Congressional Budget Office. *A Potential Influenza Pandemic: Possible Macroeconomic Effects and Policy Issues*, 8 December 2005. Accessed from website http://www.cbo.gov/showdoc.cfm?index=6946&sequence=0 on 20 December 2005.

10. Smith S. *The Economic and Social Impacts of Avian Influenza*, 12 December 2005. Accessed from website http://www.avianinfluenza.org/economic-social-impacts-avian-influenza.php on 20 December 2005.

11. Brahmbatt M. *Avian and Human Pandemic Influenza — Economic and Social Impacts*. World Bank, WHO Headquarters, Geneva, 7–9 November 2005. Accessed from website http://web.worldbank.org/WBSITE/EXTERNAL/NEWS/0,,contentMDK:20715087~pagePK:34370~piPK:42770~theSitePK:4607,00.html on 20 December 2005.

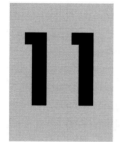

11

The Efficacy of Chinese Medicine for SARS: A Review of Important Publications from China During the Crisis

Ping-Chung Leung

Introduction

In a Chinese community, the use of Chinese medicine is common. This practice is particularly commonplace in those who suffer from poor health. When health providers and patients talk about integrated medicine or modern medicine combined with Chinese medicine, they are referring to modern treatment in complement with traditional herbal treatment — since there may never be true integration of the two systems of healing.

During the severe acute respiratory syndrome (SARS) crisis in China in 2002, there was so much uncertainty regarding the treatment of the viral pneumonia since the pathology was not clearly known and the treatment to be adopted was arbitrary. Many turned towards Chinese medicine as a supplement to the uncertain treatment. Those who were severely affected and not responding well to modern treatment naturally looked toward

Chinese medicine as an alternative. When the epidemic began to spread far and wide, healthy people immediately explored other means to prevent infection. As vaccination for the immunological protection of SARS infection was not yet available, herbal formulae became the alternative means of prevention.

The fear of infection fuelled the demand for prophylactic herbal treatment thus leading to its administration in these desperate situations, which triggered off an outcry for an "integrated approach" using both modern and traditional medicine.

When the trend spread throughout the Chinese community via the media, it moved everyone's hearts as it sparked off a cultural longing which lay dominant in every Chinese person's soul — the tradition was expected to come to the rescue of the desperate. Unchallenged accounts of the successes using traditional medicine became popular. It took no time for the belief to become prevalent and so the assumption that "integrated treatment" gave better results became widely accepted.

Now that we are facing a new threat of viral infection — the Avian Flu — which is equally unknown to us but apparently much more virulent, we should have an early exploration on the possible treatment options. If the available anti-viral or anti-flu pharmaceutical agents are not expected to be effective, alternative options become important. Alternative options used during the SARS period should be seriously assessed to get the true picture so that they can be utilized intelligently again.

Apart from general articles and media coverage on the use of traditional Chinese medicine during the SARS epidemic, there were academic reports giving details about the combined treatment from China. A critical analysis of these reports should be useful in the study of the real situation. Did Chinese medicine really help during the SARS epidemic? Did Chinese medicine reduce mortality and morbidity?

It has been known that Chinese medical professionals discussing about clinical treatments tend to be less critical compared to their counterparts reporting in the English language journals, particularly when they are dealing with clinical problems relating to Chinese medicine.[1] The failure to reach the expected depth in these clinical discussions, of course, finds its origin in the research planning and early setting of requirements. Not infrequently, Chinese medicine workers are less familiar with the conventional methodology so widely used in modern medicine. Some are not even trained to apply or understand those methodology at all.[2] When reading published reports and analyses relating to SARS treatment using Chinese medicine, one thus expects a similar type of deficiencies.

There is a myriad of literature on SARS treatment published after the SARS epidemic. An Internet search revealed a total of 130 articles. After excluding those of really poor quality, there were 90 that could be scrutinized with the aim of understanding what and how much Chinese medicine had achieved in terms of patient care.[3] We analyze the reports under three separate sections, *viz.*

(1) What the Chinese medicine practitioners claimed to have achieved?
(2) What was revealed with large-scale broad reviews on multiple reports?
(3) What herbs were used and how were these herbal preparations administered?

It is not our intention to give a detailed comprehensive analytical report, and this chapter is by no means a survey of publication statistics of facts. As a matter of fact, the emphasis and quite a number of the areas of concern of different reports were quite similar so that general reflections could be given instead of assuming that they had different messages.

By laying down the treatment facts, we hope that the actual picture during the few months of epidemic chaos would be automatically displayed. The facts were obtained from a collection of only 20 manuscripts which would be entered under the "References" section.[4,5]

What the Chinese Medicine Practitioners Claimed to have Achieved?

During the SARS period, the unanimous conclusion among the Chinese medicine practitioners was — patients treated using conventional methods fared better if also given Chinese medicine.

According to a report from Hunan province: "From a general statistical analysis, up to 20 June 2003, there were a total of 8461 cases of SARS worldwide, of which 804 died, giving an average mortality rate of 9.5%. In contrast, China reported 5326 cases of SARS with 347 dead, and a mortality rate of 6.5%. Excluding the China data, mortality rate was nearly 15%. The lower mortality rate could be attributed to the inclusion of Chinese medicine in the treatment. In fact, if only those hospitals giving integrated treatment were counted, only 28 out of 844 died, and the mortality rate was only 3.3%."

Such simple data were highly regarded without considering the possibilities of under-reporting, data confusion and imperfect categorization in China.

In fact, during the severe acute stage of SARS, all the patients should have been receiving intensive treatment regimes which might include oxygen therapy and special care: Chinese medicine practitioners would be directly involved in the treatment processes only under special circumstances. One would not be surprised that the enthusiasts built their arguments, not basing on genuine experience, but on speculations and logical thinking.[6,7]

Some reports and analysts did attempt to specify areas of concern for comparing results of treatment using conventional methods alone or combining with Chinese medicine. These areas included mortality, fever, chest radiography, steroid consumption, secondary infections, etc.[8] Other outcome measures included complications induced by steroids, remission time of symptoms of lower respiratory tract pathology (cough and shortness of breath), adverse events, laboratory parameters like loss of SARS-COV in cell cultures and PCR test, and T-lymphocyte subset counts including CD3+, CD4, CD5 and CD8.[9]

Looking at these reports which did attempt to make logical and useful observations and deductions, one readily identified the difficulties of interpretation because of the total lack of information about the timing of combined treatment, the agents used and their durations, etc. The claimed achievements of shorter time required to control a high fever, better control of symptoms like respiratory distress, smaller doses of steroidal preparations, lower mortality, better laboratory results, etc. therefore bore limited scientific significance.

What was Revealed with Large-Scale Broad Reviews on Multiple Reports?

With the obvious significance of understanding more about the claimed benefits of integrated Chinese medicine with standard hospital management, many clinicians and scientists with epidemiology background in China have made attempts to critically analyze the data expressed in a variety of published reports in different journals in China. Some of these reviews utilized the recommended methodology of system review for clinical results (Cochrane); others just tried to objectively classify the result data and compare with those that did not involve the use of Chinese medicine. Since each review involved a collection of publications and the authors did attempt to arrive at critical analysis, individual scrutiny would be performed in this chapter.

Liu *et al.* applied the established methodology of systematic review and meta analysis in a search for randomized controlled trials available from manual and electronic searches, comparing the differences between conventional treatment with combined therapy with Chinese medicine.[3]

Methodological quality of the trials was assessed by generalization of allocation sequence, allocation concealment, blinding and intention to treat.

The results showed that eight RCTs (488 patients with SARS) were
included. The methodological quality was generally low. The combined
therapy showed significant reduction of mortality (relative risk 0.32 [95%
confidence interval {CI} 0.12 to 0.91]), shortened duration of fever, symptom relief, reductions in chest radiograph abnormalities, and reductions
in secondary fungal infections among patients receiving glucocorticoids.
There were no significant effects on quality of life or glucocorticoid dosage.
The conclusion was: Chinese herbal medicine combined with conventional
medicine may have beneficial effects in patients with SARS. The evidence
is insufficient because of the low methodological quality of the included
trials.

Hao et al. from Jilin, China, selected 18 published articles for analysis.[10]
Six articles did not have a control group, three articles did not have parameters of treatment results, and all reports did not include follow-up enquiries.
The only clear observation made was that the combined treatment group
gave a lower mortality rate.

Wu et al. from the Chinese evidence-based medical center in Sichuan
province reported their review based on only nine studies which they considered qualified, in spite of uniformly obtaining serious areas of bias.[9] The
combined therapy was found to have reduced mortality, reduced fever clear-
ance time and symptom remission time. No difference was found in the
symptom scores of convalescence, cumulative doses of steroids, and inflammation resolution time.

Zhang et al., another group of epidemiologists from the same Chinese
evidence-based medical center in Sichuan, conducted their literature search
and included only six studies which fulfilled their inclusion criteria. Only
one study was graded A while five others were graded B. Results showed
only significantly better lung infiltration resorption in the combined treatment group. Mortality and cumulative doses of steroids were not found to
be different in the two groups.[11]

It seemed therefore, when individual reports were studied and analyzed,
in spite of the obvious defects, many parameters of study, e.g. mortality
or symptom controls, were found to be more positive with the combined
therapy group. However, when more reports were reviewed together, it
became more difficult to acquire more convincing evidence.

If blood results could be taken as more objective and were subjected to
less bias when results were assessed, one observation could be made. Many
reports did show less reduction of the T-lymphocyte subsets of CD3, CD4

and CD5, and others which might be supportive of the immuno-supportive nature of some herbal formulae and compounds.[12,13]

What Herbs were Used and How were These Herbal Preparations Administered?

The advocates of herbal treatment and combined therapy would of course be keen to give details of the therapy, including the commodities of herbs utilized. Analytic accounts of the herbal preparations used for different symptoms and syndrome complexes were also given. Thus, specific herbal treatment targeting against specific symptoms included the following: fever, thirst, cough, sputum, shortness of breadth, sweating, sleeplessness, nausea, poor appetite, hemoptysis, bowel disturbance, urinary disturbances, tightness of chest, abdominal discomfort, limb weakness, headache and faintness.[14]

Chinese herbalists prescribe according to general syndrome complexes known to the profession as conventional rules guiding the individualization of treatment. Herbal experts participating in the combined treatment also prescribe according to the syndrome complexes and a summary is given in Table 1.[6]

Some reports gave long lists of herbal choices including individual ones, classical formulae with or without innovative modifications and proprietor preparations, which might have been derived from classic formulae or were from modern Chinese medicinal products.[4]

In spite of the attempts to correlate the treatment of various syndromes with special choices, there were so many duplications that the experience had not been too meaningful as future references. One interesting attempt was made to divide the SARS infection into four stages, *viz.* early, middle, late and rehabilitation, and thence, tried to identify the popular choices during each individual stage. The aim might have been the establishment of a systematic documentation for future reference. This attempt again, because of the massive duplications, could not have been too realistic.[4]

Isolated reports on the endorsement and advocation of certain specific formulation or proprietor preparation for either general SARS treatment or specific syndrome complex related to the disease were also found.[15] The objectivity and true value of such isolated reports should be doubted.

One article in the *China Journal of Chinese Materia Medica* gave a valuable account of the different state/provincial level recommendations of herbal treatment during the different stages of SARS infection. Responsible

Table 1: The herbs prescribed by Chinese herbalists for various syndrome complexes.

Syndrome complex	Herbal name	Pharmacological effects						Use	
		Anti-viral / Anti-bacterial	Anti-heating?	Immuno-boosting / Anti-allergy	Anti-inflammation	Anti-fibrosis	Improve circulation	Prevention	Treatment according to (staging)
Sick feeling	Radix Bupleuri	+/+	+	+/	+			+	Early
	Radix Saposhnikoviae	+/+	+	+/	+			+	Early
	Herba Schizonepetae	/+	+	/+	+		+	+	Early
	Folium Perillae	+	+					+	Early
	Flos Chrysanthemi	+/+	+				+	+	Early
Toxic heat	Fructus Forsythiae	+/+	+		+			+	Early
	Herba Houttuyniae	+/+		/+	+	+			Early, middle
	Radix Isatidis	+/+		+/				+	Middle
	Rhizoma Cibotii	+/-						+	
	Rhizoma Dryopteris Crassirhizomae	+/						+	
Osmunda japonica Thunb.	Osnum Cyntonium	+/							Early
	Radix Scutellariae	+/+	+	+/+	+		+	+	Early, middle
	Rhizoma Belamcandae	+/+	+	+	+			+	Early
	Herba Erodii/ Herba Geranii	+/+						+	Early
	Rhizoma Fagopyri Dibotryis	/+	+	++	+				Early, middle

Table 1: (*Continued*)

Syndrome complex	Herbal name	Anti-viral Anti-bacterial	Anti-heating?	Immuno-boosting/ Anti-allergy	Anti-inflammation	Anti-fibrosis	Improve circulation	Prevention	Use: Treatment according to (staging)
Trollius chinensis Bge.	*Trollius chinensis* Bge.	/ +							Early
	Flos Lonicerae	+/+	+	+/+	+			+	Early
	Gypsum Fibrosum		+				+		Early, middle, late
	Cornu Saigae Tataricae		+						Middle
Humid	Rhizoma Atractylodis	+/+		+				+	Rehabilitation
Eupatorium fortunei Turcz.	Herbra Eupatorii	+/		+				+	Early
	Herba Agastachis	+/+					+	+	Early
	Semen Coicis	/+		+/	+			+	
Rheumatic	Rhizoma Polygoni Cuspidati	+/+					+		Middle, rehabilitation
Bowel obstruction	Radix et Rhizoma Rhei	+/+	+		+				Late
Circulatory stagnation	Radix Salviae Miltiorrhizae	+/+		+/	+	+	+		Late
	Herba Erigerontis	+/+				+	+		Middle, late
	Stigma Croci				+		+		Late

Table 1: (*Continued*)

Syndrome complex	Herbal name	Pharmacological effects						Use	
		Anti-viral Anti-bacterial	Anti-heating?	Immuno-boosting/ Anti-allergy	Anti-inflammation	Anti-fibrosis	Improve circulation	Prevention	Treatment according to (staging)
Deficiency	Radix Pseudostellariae			+/			+		Rehabilitation
	Radix Panacis Quinquefolii		+				+		Rehabilitation
	Radix Astragali	+/+		+/	+		+	+	Early
	Radix Glycyrrhizae	+/+		+/+	+			+	Early
	Rhizoma Atractylodis Macrocephalae	/+			+			+	Rehabilitation
Dryness	Fructus Schisandrae Chinensis	+/			+				Rehabilitation
Feeling empty	Herba Dendrobii		+	+/			+		Rehabilitation
	Radix Ophiopogonis	+/		+/+			+		Rehabilitation
Feeling deficient	Radix Rehmanniae			+/+	+		+		Late, rehabilitation
Chesty and phlamy	Radix Platycodonis	/+			+				Early

organizations included the Guangdong Chinese Medicine Control Bureau, giving the Guangdong recommendation; the Beijing Center of Command for SARS treatment, giving the Beijing recommendation; the State Chinese Medicine Bureau and Health Department, giving the National Recommendation; and the Science and Technology Division, Health Department and State Chinese Medicine Bureau, giving eight preparations for SARS treatment.[16] A summary of the varieties of recommendations are given in Table 2.

There was a general belief that Chinese medicine was mild, and was suitable for all, while adverse effects were negligible. The SARS crisis was such an important era that even enthusiasts critically looked at the treatment processes. When herbal combinations were used, adverse effects were areas of particular concern. Chi in Shanxi reviewed over 2000 cases of herbal consumption in hospitals and clinics and identified 163 cases (5%–6%) of adverse effects. Details of the adverse effects were given in Table 3.[17]

Table 2: Recommendations of herbal treatment during the different SARS infection stages.

Recommended prescription	Origin	Indication	Number of herbs
1	Guang Dong	Early stage	11
2	Guang Dong	Early stage	9
3	Guang Zhou	Middle stage	14
4	Guang Zhou	Middle stage	9
5	Guang Zhou	Middle stage	12
6	Guang Zhou	Late stage	5
7	Guang Zhou	Late stage	2
8	Guang Zhou	Rehabilitation stage	8
9	Guang Zhou	Rehabilitation stage	12
10	Beijing	Suspected	13
11	Beijing	High fever	11
12	Beijing	Cough	11
13	Beijing	Rehabilitation stage	12
14	National Bureau	Prevention	5
15	National Bureau	Prevention	5
16	National Bureau	Prevention	5
17	National Bureau	Prevention	5
18	National Bureau	Prevention	8
19	National Bureau	Prevention	10
20	National Bureau	Mild services	12
21	National Bureau	Serious services	11
22	National Bureau	Rehabilitation stage	12
23	Qing Kai Ling	All types	7
24	Sin Sui Granules	High fever	8

Table 3: Adverse effects caused by herbal combinations.

Category	Group A (Severe)	Group B (Mild)	Total
Rash	1	22	23
Erythematous rash	4	13	17
Fluctuating erythema	6	12	18
Erythema	2	14	16
Exfoliative dermatitis	0	4	4
Anaphylactic purpura	0	10	10
Multiple eczema	0	19	19
Laryngeal oedema	0	2	2
Respiratory distress	0	2	2
Palpitation	0	3	3
Abdominal pain	0	14	14
Diarrhea	2	24	26
Anaphylactic shock	0	1	1
Liver dysfunction	0	3	3
Abnormal ECG	0	1	1
Proteinuria	0	2	2
Total	17	146	163

Why is a Proper Review of the Results of Integrated Treatment for the SARS Victims Important?

Today, the causative agent for SARS is clear. It was the coronavirus that was responsible for a series of pathological events which threaten the normal functioning of the infected. The virus first caused a short period of flu-like symptoms, then produced excessive inflammatory reactions in the respiratory system resulting in respiratory distress. The excessive inflammatory responses needed to be suppressed with steroidal management which would cut down tissue responses and exudations. If herbal treatment really helped, either in the acute stage of inflammation which hopefully could have been suppressed, or during the steroidal stage when the dependence on the steroidal suppression of inflammation could have been alleviated, the future treatment for viral pneumonia would have to be rewritten. Since herbal treatment is most probably multi-targeted and seldom specific, what was observed during the SARS period might be repeated for any respiratory tract infection caused by viral factors, bearing a similar symptomatology. The herbal preparations utilized during the SARS crisis were based on classical records treating diseases that resembled the symptomatology of flu and respiratory distress. If the traditional formulae did help in the SARS crisis, they should also help in any future flu or bird flu epidemic.[18]

A critical look at the reports available, including those that directly nar-
rated the experience, claiming impressive results, and those analyzing the
reported results, gave no convincing account of the effectiveness, but only
indications of probable effects on improving the fatality and controlling
some of the symptoms.

One should not be disappointed with the observations of limited value.
Rather, a sensible future policy should be worked out based on the valuable
observations.

Discussion

Whether the 2002 SARS epidemic originated in the Pearl Delta of the
Guangdong province of China or elsewhere was not entirely clear. However, that the first case of SARS in China occurred in the Pearl Delta region,
and which later spread to Guangzhou, Hong Kong and Beijing was an
officially accepted fact. It was observed that the mortality rate of SARS in
China was apparently lower than those in other countries, including Hong
Kong, Toronto and Singapore. It had been revealed in the media, throughout the SARS outbreak, that Chinese physicians were applying an integrated
approach, using both modern medicine and herbs, in the treatment of SARS.
It was, therefore, assumed that this integrated approach had brought down
the mortality rate.

The Chinese Center for Disease Control and Prevention under the Ministry of Health, China, issued special instructions and guidelines to the
hospitals and clinics on special disease conditions and their diagnoses and
treatments. Such guidelines were quite specific and detailed. In April 2003,
the center gathered all the available information from both within and outside China, gave an updated analysis, and revised the deduction on the
SARS outbreak. A complete set of documents, containing details of etiology, diagnostic criteria, clinical manifestations, management, instructions,
drugs used, preventive means and Chinese medicinal considerations was
produced.

Concerning Chinese medicine, the center labeled SARS as a form of Wan
Bing (溫病). Wan Bing, meaning diseases with temperature, was an important
specialization within traditional Chinese medicine. Although diseases with
increased body temperature were described and well documented more
than 2000 years ago in the Han Dynasty, when Zhang Zhon-jing (張仲景), one
of the forefathers of Chinese medicine, wrote his book "Shang-han Luen"
(傷寒論), and although the classic volume had been taken as a detailed documentation on typhoid, the descriptions in reality, exceeded the realm of

typhoid. It encompassed a much larger area of diseases of probably infectious nature. Followers of Zhang refined and expanded the understanding
of the specialty during the dynasties following Han. A clear-cut and well-
recognized specialty of Wan Bing finally matured in the years between the
Ming and Qing Dynasties. It is not an exaggeration to consider this specialty as the most important branch of Chinese herbal medicine, covering
the most frequently encountered areas of the herbalist's practice, command-
ing numerous volumes of case reports and prescriptions, and above all, it
has been included in the teaching curricula of all educational set-ups on
Chinese medicine and is considered mandatory.

A term coined using the common language of everyday use, Wan Bing
was understood as referring to the common, feverish diseases appearing
at the intervals between weather changes, i.e. between spring and summer,
and between autumn and winter. These feverish diseases were contagious,
first spreading within the family household, later spreading outside to the
village; and later, even across villages.

Having labeled the current SARS outbreak as a form of Wan Bing, the
Chinese Center for Disease Control and Prevention recommended treatment protocols, according to the Wan Bing classical teaching. With regard
to hospitalized patients, the center's guidelines for treatment include the
following:

(1) use antibiotics to prevent bacterial infection,
(2) consider using steroidal preparations to control excessive immunological responses,
(3) consider using herbal preparations as an adjuvant therapy, and
(4) use antiviral preparations.[19]

From the official national guidelines on the treatment of SARS, it
was obvious that as far as hospitalized patients were concerned, modern
medicine remained the mainstream treatment and Chinese medicine was
used as a supportive adjuvant therapy. There were no instructions on the
use of herbal medicine in the management of SARS during the early, pre-
hospitalized stage or the later convalescent, rehabilitation stage.

One has to understand that although some hospitals in China were
named "Chinese Medicine Hospital," it does not mean that only Chinese
medicine is prescribed as the agent for healing. In fact, the so-called Chinese
Medicine Hospitals fulfill the duties of any other hospitals, i.e. catering
to emergencies, intensive care and invasive means of rescue, like modern investigations, surgeries and other interventions. The only difference,

unique to Chinese Medicine Hospital, is that Chinese medicine use is most frequently considered, whenever treatment is being offered. When SARS patients were admitted into Chinese Medicine Hospitals, therefore, herbal medicine would be used as part of the treatment regime. As for the other hospitals, whether Chinese medicine would be included as an adjuvant therapy, would depend on the preferences of the attending team of physicians and the patients and their relatives. Only about 10% of the hospitals in China carried the hallmark of Chinese Medicine Hospital and were functionally Chinese Medicine Hospitals.

Based on these facts, an estimated 40%–60% of hospitalized SARS patients at some stage of their treatment, received an integrated approach, combining both modern and Chinese medicine. This was confirmed by the Deputy Minister of Health of Municipal Beijing towards the end stage of the SARS outbreak.

Positive reports, during the SARS epidemic, were quite plentiful. A professor from Shanghai visited the Chinese Medicine University in Guangzhou in early June 2003, and reported that the first affiliated hospital of the University treated 60 patients with SARS, and the mortality rate was zero. The second affiliated hospital treated double the number of SARS patients, and the mortality rate was only 6%, well below the data known for SARS infection outside China. Furthermore, it was reported that the hospital workers took prophylactic herbal drinks and none of them fell sick in spite of the high risk nature of their job.

More detailed information about the treatment regimes was revealed in a teleconference between Taiwanese experts and Beijing physicians during the peak of the outbreak in Taiwan. Apart from emphasizing the effectiveness of herbal medicine as an adjuvant therapy for SARS patients, and the need to properly utilize oxygen therapy, respirators and steroids, a number of injection solutions manufactured from herbs were recommended to facilitate rapid interventional supplements. They were Qing Kai Ling (清開靈), a proprietor injection preparation; Herba Houttuyniae (魚腥草); Radix Isatidis (板藍根); and Xiangdian (香丹), another proprietor mixture.

As prophylaxis, six prescriptions were given.[20] They were

(1) Formula 1: Radix Astragali (黃蓍), Herba Patriniae (敗醬草),
                Semen Coicis (薏苡仁), Radix Platycodonis (桔梗), and
                Radix Glycyrrhizae (生甘草).
(2) Formula 2: Herba Houttuyniae (魚腥草), Flos Chrysanthemi Indici
                (野菊花), Herba Artemisiae Scopariae (茵陳),
                Eupatorium Fortunei (佩蘭), and Fructus Tsaoko (草果).

(3) Formula 3: Herba Taraxaci (蒲公英), Trollius Chinensis Bge (金蓮花), Folium Isatidis (大青葉), Radix Puerariae (葛根), and Folium Perillae (蘇葉).

(4) Formula 4: Rhizoma Phragmitis (蘆根), Flos Lonicerae (銀花), Fructus Forsythiae (連翹), Herba Menthae (薄荷), and Radix Glycyrrhizae (生甘草).

(5) Formula 5: Radix Astragali (黃蓍), Rhizoma Atractylodis Macrocephalae (白朮), Radix Saposhnikoviae (防風), Rhizoma Atractylodis (蒼朮), Herba Agastachis (藿香), Adenophora Verticillata (沙參), Flos Lonicerae (銀花), and Rhizoma Dryopteris Crassirhizomae (綿馬貫眾).

(6) Formula 6: Radix Pseudostellariae (太子參), Rhizoma Dryopteris Crassirhizomae (綿馬貫眾), Flos Lonicerae (銀花), Fructus Forsythiae (連翹), Folium Isatidis (大青葉), Folium Perillae (蘇葉), Radix Puerariae (葛根), Herba Agastachis (藿香), Rhizoma Atractylodis (蒼朮), and Eupatorium Fortunei (佩蘭).

Wan Bing was interpreted as a seasonal disease related to changing of the weather, particularly before and during early summer. The Wan Bing philosophy advocates protection against falling ill as the weather turns increasingly warm and becoming unbearable, or when the reverse is happening during autumn. With this traditional belief, every household in the Chinese community, under the care of senior members, would prepare favorable fruits, soups and herbal drinks to "clear" the heat. When one family member starts running a fever, all members are given the same herbal drink to arrest further development.

What are the Herbs Used?

The influence of the Wan Bing school of thought is so wide and real that simple "anti-fever" formulae and their derivatives have been most commonly known and used for decades. During the SARS outbreak, people in Hong Kong and the mainland used many different herbal preparations in an attempt to protect against getting infected.

Some time in late February 2003, when the outbreak around the Pearl Delta was at its peak, citizens and villagers boiled vinegar to generate an acidic steam to fumigate their households. This practice apparently dated back to centuries ago (might be medieval) and whether it did control any viral spread was never proven. Nevertheless, one fringe benefit of this practice must be the increase in the awareness within the community of the existence of a contagious disease.

The course of events in a SARS patient followed quite closely that of the much more familiar influenza, *viz.* feverishness, fever, malaise, muscle aches, chills, cough, shortness of breath and pneumonia. The main differences lie in the speed of infection and the apparently much higher incidence of pneumonia among the SARS victims.

Wan Bing scholars had different ways of defining the course of events, relying on the severity and behavior of the affected patient. The best established theory could simply be described in four terms: Wai (衛), Qi (氣), Yin (營) and Zhur (血), which have been interpreted either as the stages of clinical manifestation or alternatively, the different principles of management at different stages of clinical manifestation. In the former context, Wai and Qi might mean early onset of feverishness and running nose; Yin and Zhur might mean deterioration of respiratory symptoms ending in hemoptysis. In the latter context of understanding, Wai-Qi is a therapeutic approach whereby the Qi needs to be protected; and later, as the disease progresses, the Zhur component, i.e. the real essence of vitality, is being challenged and hence requires laborious support.

If Chinese medicine works well for Wan Bing, which is related to either influenza or contagious diseases of the respiratory system, one might have little hesitation using herbal remedy during the early stages of influenza, perhaps including SARS, when life support and other specific treatments are not yet required. It is therefore logical to suggest that, Chinese medicine could be seriously considered as a treatment option during the early stages of viral infections affecting the respiratory tract, but should play only a supporting role when the disease progresses. Modern medications like antibiotics and other more specific items like steroids, should not be given at the early stages, but should be administered only when observations confirmed the seriousness of the disease and their use is clearly indicated. Using Chinese herbal preparations at the observational stages, therefore, could be a logical practical supplement.

During the SARS epidemic, in spite of the wide media coverage that integrated modern treatment with traditional Chinese medicine, in attempts to better serve the victims, had achieved a lot: from lowering the mortality rates to the better control of symptoms like respiratory stress and the reduction of steroidal dosages, there were no convincing indications that the reports were scientifically trustworthy. While one realizes that under the stress of the epidemic, any evidence-based trial with logical planning would not have been feasible, one should still rely on available information to judge whether Chinese medicine did help. One positive observation was that there were neither reports about serious adverse effects of herbal medicine during the SARS period nor suggestions that herbal treatment interfered with conventional modern treatment. The available data only showed that Chinese medicine, during the crisis, was never seriously used as the mainline treatment, but instead was often used as a formal adjunct to the mainline treatment. Chinese medicine was used as a supplement to the measures of symptomatic control. Indeed some distinguished physicians in China understood such use as the "conceptual" use of Chinese medicine. A proper review of the available literature should help to stop the prevalent observation (or assumption) that Chinese medicine worked so well during one viral respiratory infection crisis, therefore it should also work well and should be very much advocated in an expected future viral attack. Rather, the issue of supplementing mainline treatment with Chinese medicine, should be seriously looked into, put into practical research contexts using scientific methodology in its proper objective evaluation. Early treatment or prevention should attract genuine attention and interests.

In fact, once a patient suffering from viral infection affecting the respiratory tract is admitted into a hospital, respiratory distress or severe life-threatening symptoms like hyperpyrexia or other medical complications are expected. The mainline approach to such a situation, should therefore, be emergency medicine or target-orientated treatment, which Chinese medicine has relatively little to offer. Chinese medicine treatment in the hospital therefore, would need to remain supportive.

Indeed, one important publication after the SARS crises summarized the total drug expenditure in the Beijing Xiao Tang Shan Hospital, which was built as an emergency measure to accommodate over 680 SARS patients. The statistics given by the dispensary indicated that the majority of the drugs used belonged to the mainline modern medicine preparations, whereas only a small proportion belonged to various Chinese medicine categories, a lot of which were of proprietor nature. The indications of use were mainly for the control of symptoms like cough, high fever and diarrhea.[21]

A realistic analysis of the factual data during the SARS crisis did indicate a supportive role rather than a crucial role of Chinese medicine in the hospital settings. This understanding should not have undermined the value of Chinese medicine for the treatment of viral diseases affecting the respiratory tract. There is always an early stage of viral infection when symptoms are mild and not affecting the lungs. Classics in Chinese medicine offer much evidence of the value of Chinese medicine as we have already discussed.

Early treatment refers to symptoms of feverishness and malaise before the respiratory distress symptoms actually arrive. What about even before these early symptoms? If the individual uses Chinese medicine at the earliest feeling of affection, would it not be equivalent to a prophylactic manoeuvre? Is there a role for Chinese medicine to be used as a prophylactic or preventive measure? Is the preventive measure a recognized concept?

During the SARS crisis, vigorous debate did occur among distinguished Chinese medicine experts in China. The debate involved two opposing parties: those supporting the household use of prophylactic Chinese medicine and those bitterly attacking the concept as wasting resources and might be producing confusing pictures and even unnecessary adverse effects.[22]

In fact, as early as 3000 years ago, it was recorded in the most ancient classical writing of medicine, Su-Wen (素問), that one herbal formula might suit a lot of people. Some distinguished experts on Wan Bing also wrote that when the feverish epidemic affected large districts and populations, there should be the understanding that simple, uniform herbal formula might have to be used for all. In such a situation, the important Chinese medicine principle of individualization of treatment program, could be dropped.[23]

Now that we are expecting an epidemic, or even a pandemic of avian flu, what we have learned from the SARS crisis should be good reference to our plan for the immediate future. Interesting results were obtained, using Chinese medicine as a preventive agent against SARS infection.

At the peak of the SARS epidemic in Hong Kong, hospital workers were under high risks of contraction of the infection. Herbal preparations had been used historically in China to treat influenza-like diseases. During the SARS outbreak, herbal preparations had been used jointly with standard modern treatment in China. As a means to protect the at-risk hospital workers, an innovative herbal formula was created and consumed by 3160 of them in two weeks. During the two weeks, symptoms and adverse effects were closely monitored; 37 of them had their serum checked for immunological responses.

The results showed that none of the herb consumers contracted the infection, compared to 0.4% among the non-consumers. Adverse effects had been infrequent and mild. There were hardly any influenza-like symptoms and the quality of life improved. In the group who volunteered to have their immunological state checked, significant boosting effects were found. It was concluded that there might be a good indication for using suitable herbal preparations as a means of preventing influenza-like infection. The mode of preventive effect could be treatment of the infection at its very early stage instead of producing a period of higher immunological ability, as in the case of vaccination.[24]

While the creation of an effective vaccine would be the most logical solution to the problem of any new infection, the difficulties already encountered for AIDS and Influenza are valuable reminders that science, in the strictly conventional sense, might take time for maturation. Hence, before the day that the viral respiratory infection could be completely brought under control using science, like vaccine creation, there is a place for the exploration of other means, like herbal alternative medicine, in the treatment, and particularly, in the prevention of frank infection developing into pneumonia.

References

1. Tang JL, Zhau SY, Ernst E. Review of randomised controlled trials of traditional Chinese medicine. *Br Med J* 1999;819:161.
2. Klemman A. *Medicine in Chinese Culture: Comparative Studies of Healthcare in China and Other Countries*. US Department of Health, Education and Welfare, Washington DC, 1975; Centre for Disease Control and Prevention, Ministry of Health, China.
3. Liu J, Manheimer E, Shi Y, *et al.* Chinese herbal medicine for severe acute respiratory syndrome: a systematic review and meta-analysis. *J Altern Complement Med* 2004;10(6):1041–1051.
4. Shao KL, Sung K, Yuen CJ, *et al.* Literature review of stage treatment of SARS using principles of Chinese medicine. *J Tradit Chin Med Univ Hunan* 2005;25(2):53–55.
5. Wang ZM, Zhu XX, Cui XL, *et al.* Screening of traditional Chinese remedies for SARS treatment. *China J Chin Mater Med* 2003;28(6):484–487.
6. Shao PG, Wang YY, Chen HS. Clues on the use of Chinese medicine for the treatment of SARS. *China J Chin Mater Med* 2003;28(6):481–483.
7. Zhao CH, Guo YB, Wu H, *et al.* Clinical manifestation, treatment, and outcome of severe acute respiratory syndrome: analysis of 108 cases in Beijing. *Natl Med J China* 2003;83(11):897–901.
8. Lin L, Xu YJ, He DP, *et al.* A retrospective study on clinical features of and treatment methods for 77 severe cases of SARS. *Am J Chin Med* 2003;31(6):821–839.
9. Wu TX, Liu BY, Liu GJ, *et al.* A systematic review of assessing the effect of integrated traditional Chinese medicine with Western medicine for severe acute respiratory syndrome. *Chin J Evid Based Med* 2004;4(4):226–238.
10. Hao YK, Hung J, Kao CK. Meta-analysis of SARS treatment using integrated medicine. *Chin J Public Health* 2005;21(5):525–526.

11. Zhang MM, Liu XM, He L, *et al.* Effect of integrated traditional Chinese and Western medicine on SARS: a review of clinical evidence. *World J Gastroenterol* 2004;10(23):3500–3505.

12. Zheng X, Cai C, Huang Y, *et al.* Analyses of subset, activated state and expression pattern of 24 repertoire TCR Vß of peripheral blood T lymphocytes in convalescence patients with severe acute respiratory syndrome (SARS). *Chin J Cell Mol Immunol* 2005;21(1):114–117.

13. Csi C, Zeng X, Ou AH, *et al.* The study on T cell subsets and their activated molecules from the convalescent SARS patients during two follow-up surveys. *Chin J Cell Mol Immunol* 2004;20(3):322–324.

14. Li SW, Hu JH, Yang Y, *et al.* Analysis of 63 cases of SARS presenting with Chinese medicine syndromes. *China J Integr Tradit West Med* 2003;23(8):569–571.

15. Cai L, Zhang TC, Zhang M. Efficacy of compound glycyrrhizic acid in treatment of SARS. *Chin J New Drugs* 2004;13(9):842–845.

16. Shao SH, Wang JB, Hor CS. Analysis of Chinese medicine formulae used for SARS treatment. *China J Chin Mater Med* 2003;28(7):664–668.

17. Qi WS. Adverse effects of Chinese medicine used for SARS treatment. *China J Chin Med Inf* 2003;10(12):39–40.

18. Leung PC. Herbal medicine in the treatment of SARS. In: *Severe Acute Respiratory Syndrome: From Benchtop to Bedside* (ed.) Sung JJY. World Scientific Publishing Co., Singapore, 2003, pp. 184–202.

19. Treatment of SARS (http://www.satcm.gov.cn/lanmu/feidian/030529/liangan.htm).

20. Instructions on the treatment of SARS (http://www.satcm.gov.cn/lanmu/feidian/tcm030606jieshao.htm).

21. Wang R, Zhou XQ, Dong J, *et al.* Utilization analysis of drug efficacy of the 680 cases of SARS patients in Xiao Tang Shan Hospital of PLA. *Chin J Evid Based Med* 2004;4(7):474–481.

22. Liu BY. *SARS Treatment — The Beijing Experience.* SARS Conference, Polytechnic University, 14 July 2003.

23. Bian YJ, Qi WS, Song QQ, *et al.* Evaluation on effect of integrative medical treatment on quality of life of rehabilitation stage in 85 patients with SARS. *Chin J Integr Tradit West Med* 2003;23(9):658–660.

24. Lau JTF, Leung PC, Wong ELY, *et al.* The use of an herbal formula by hospital care workers during the severe acute respiratory syndrome epidemic in Hong Kong to prevent severe acute respiratory syndrome transmission, relieve influenza-related symptoms, and improve quality of life: a prospective cohort study. *J Altern Complement Med* 2005;11(1):49–55.

12

Scientific, Organizational and Economic Issues in Pandemic Influenza Vaccine Development

Vincent T.-K. Chow

This chapter on pandemic influenza vaccine development is framed as frequently asked questions with corresponding responses based on existing scientific evidence and/or considered projections of opinion leaders. The discussion points are by no means comprehensive and final due to the constantly changing dynamics of the H5N1 avian influenza virus and its continuing spread among animals and humans. In addition to influenza immunization, more research also needs to be conducted to gain a better understanding of influenza virus biology, virus-host interactions, and mechanisms of antiviral drug resistance.[1]

What are the Influenza Vaccines Currently in Use?

Infections with influenza viruses are common among humans, and pose health risks among certain groups of people which may result in serious or life-threatening complications.

There are two types of vaccines for immunization against human influenza. The inactivated vaccine containing killed virus is administered by injection, and is approved for use in individuals over six months of age, including healthy persons and those with chronic diseases. The nasal-spray vaccine is produced with live but weakened influenza viruses, and is approved for healthy persons aged five to 49 years without pre-existing medical problems and who are not pregnant.

Due to the propensity of influenza viruses to mutate, vaccines are produced every year against various strains of human influenza, and have a shelf-life of about six months. Typically, the vaccine contains three strains, i.e. two belonging to influenza virus type A (e.g. H1N1 and H3N2), and one type B strain. The strains in the vaccine are selected on the basis of international surveillance and estimations by scientists on the predominant virus types and strains that circulate in a particular year. Thus, the composition of the seasonal influenza vaccines may differ for the winter periods in the northern and southern hemispheres. For example, in 2005, one of the three influenza strains in the northern hemisphere vaccine differed significantly from the southern hemisphere vaccine.

The single best way to protect against influenza is to get immunized before winter in temperate countries. In the northern hemisphere, the optimal time for vaccination is October to December, i.e. at or before the beginning of the flu season which may start in October and end in May. It should be emphasized that the efficacy of the vaccine is dependent on its being current, and one should ensure that the vaccine received is up to date. About two weeks after immunization, antibodies that confer protection against the specific vaccine strains develop in the vaccinated individual (vaccinee).

Can Current Flu Vaccines Protect Against Bird Flu?

Conventional flu vaccines only provide protection against the common strains of human influenza. So far, there is no evidence to show that current seasonal flu vaccines protect humans against H5N1 avian influenza.

It is important to note that flu vaccines are not required for the general population. Vaccination against human influenza is recommended for persons who are at higher risk of developing complications from influenza, such as pneumonia. The high-risk group comprises the elderly over 65 years of age, children, people with chronic heart and lung diseases (including asthma), chronic metabolic diseases (including diabetes mellitus), kidney dysfunction, immune suppression, and women in the second or third trimester of pregnancy.

Although flu vaccines do not offer protection against the deadly H5N1 virus, they reduce opportunities for dual infections. Scientists fear that a mutant flu strain that triggers a human pandemic may arise from recombination between human and bird flu strains in dually infected cells.

Are Vaccines Against Pandemic Bird Flu Necessary?

Influenza viruses constantly mutate at random resulting in seasonal influenza. However, these viruses may undergo major genetic changes that enable them to rapidly infect and kill millions of people in catastrophic global pandemics. For example, a deadly mutant flu strain that "jumps" from animals to humans can spark a severe pandemic.

During the 20th century, three flu pandemics caused severe disease, not only among the susceptible young and elderly groups, but also in other healthy individuals. The "Spanish flu" pandemic of 1918–1919 was the most notorious and devastating epidemic in recorded history, which affected one-quarter of the world's population and killed between 40 and 50 million people, i.e. more deaths than World War I itself.[2] This pandemic preceded the discovery of penicillin and other antibiotics, and occurred before modern air travel with its fleets of airplanes connecting many parts of the world. Although the 1957 "Asian flu" and 1968 "Hong Kong flu" pandemics were considered milder, they killed three million people worldwide.

More recently, in 1997 and 2003, the new H5N1 subtype of influenza A virus emerged in Asia, culminating in direct transmission from infected birds to humans with lethal consequences. Notwithstanding the unprecedented efforts to limit their spread, H5N1 viruses have continued their relentless march within and outside Asia, and have expanded their reach into the European and African continents. In September 2004, the Food and Agriculture Organization and the World Organization for Animal Health warned that bird flu is endemic in Asia, and constitutes a crisis of global importance as well as a permanent threat to animal and human health.

Although bird flu is currently transmitted from infected animals to people, there are worries that the H5N1 strain may randomly mutate or combine with a human influenza strain and acquire the ability to spread easily among humans, triggering a worldwide pandemic. Interestingly, a previous study suggests that the bird flu virus may already have been transmitted among humans without signs of illness. Although some health care workers did not manifest any symptoms during the 1997 outbreak in Hong Kong, they had antibodies to bird flu virus, implying sub-clinical infection acquired from their patients.[3]

Many virologists believe that a global outbreak of pandemic influenza is overdue. Will a similar modern pathogen reproduce another monumental global disaster like the 1918 pandemic? Will the devastation be magnified by mass global travel? Will advances in medicine and biology, new antiviral innovations, and global preparedness plans offer real hope to contain the threat? For the moment, we have no answers to these troubling questions.

No one can predict when or where a lethal flu strain that is highly contagious among humans will emerge. Due to modern travel trends, another pandemic could strike within months or even weeks. Given the gravity of the threat, it would be irresponsible not to prepare and be ready for a worst-case scenario. In such a situation, it is not inconceivable that hospital services would be overwhelmed, riots would wreak havoc at clinics, while food and power shortages would occur.

Officials have warned that even developed countries such as the US are ill-equipped to contain or control a new influenza pandemic. No time should be wasted to start planning adequate preparatory countermeasures to confront a potential disaster.[4] Such a broad contingency plan will require immediate resources and extensive coordinated efforts by governments as well as national and international agencies. The response plan to deal with a pandemic would include rapid diagnostic test kits, reliable surveillance systems, travel restrictions, quarantine, stockpiling and administration of anti-influenza drugs.[5–7]

Although a few antiviral drugs have been used against H5N1, some strains have developed resistance to amantadine. Deaths of two bird flu patients in Vietnam attributed to oseltamivir (tamiflu) resistance have also raised concerns.[8] Indiscriminate use of antiviral drugs is expected to result in the inevitable appearance and escalation of drug-resistant flu viruses.

Since humans lack immunity to the H5N1 strain, the ideal protection is an effective vaccine. As an alternative to biosecurity, the rapid development and subsequent utilization of pandemic influenza vaccines are therefore necessary and needed urgently.[9] The World Health Organization (WHO) is actively working with member nations and industry to address the need to produce vastly increased quantities of vaccine to counter a potential pandemic. In September 2004, WHO convened a meeting of pharmaceutical industry representatives, and urged them to intensify efforts to boost vaccine manufacturing capacity. Should a pandemic suddenly erupt, it may be possible to dampen the first wave of infections by initially deploying antiviral agents. Moreover, if the pandemic strain can be rushed into an emergency plan to produce and administer vaccines quickly enough, the second wave of infections may possibly be further attenuated.[10]

What are the Technologies for Producing Flu Vaccines?

Because flu viruses mutate so quickly, flu vaccines must be prepared fresh annually. Each year, the three strains expected to be the most prevalent for the flu season are inoculated and replicated in fertilized chicken eggs, before a long process of chemical inactivation and packaging. Influenza vaccines thus rely on the standard system of growth in millions of chicken eggs, take about nine months to produce, and do not confer optimal protection. This conventional practice of making flu vaccines is decades old and has changed little, entailing a production process that is cumbersome, inflexible and uncertain. Such a system poses a huge problem because vaccines are biological products which cannot be generated rapidly in large quantities should a flu pandemic erupt.

Unfortunately, the egg technology does not work for the lethal H5N1 because this strain kills the developing chick embryo before sufficient amounts of virus can be harvested. To circumvent this, a technique known as reverse genetic engineering can be exploited to alter the genetics of the strain to facilitate its growth in eggs.[11,12] As part of flu pandemic planning, the US Department of Health and Human Services has contracted Sanofi-Aventis and Chiron to prepare batches of vaccine using reverse genetics. The product is a hybrid consisting of a standard flu vaccine strain that incorporates genes derived from an H5N1 strain isolated from a Vietnamese patient in 2004.

Most government and pharmaceutical efforts are seeking to develop better technologies to manufacture flu vaccines more rapidly, to accelerate advances to deliver the next generation of vaccine production technology.[13] US President George W. Bush has requested Congress for US$7.1 billion in emergency funding to combat influenza, of which US$2.8 billion has been assigned to replace the dated egg-based vaccine process. Instead of using eggs, experts agree that the best strategy is cell-based vaccine production which is easier to handle, and involves culturing the virus for producing vaccines in batches of human or mammalian cells in the laboratory. Recent seasonal flu vaccine shortages, the extraordinary geographical spread of the H5N1 virus, and the potential emergence of a new deadly pandemic strain have made the need for this faster method even more pressing.[14]

DNA vaccines represent a potentially simpler and more rapid approach for producing vaccines within three months, and do not require chicken eggs. This strategy involves the cloning of specific virus genes and injecting the DNA into humans. Should the flu virus mutate significantly, scientists can isolate and clone relevant genes from the mutant strain to generate new vaccines. Such vaccines have proven successful in mice,[15] while limited clinical trials with improved versions and protocols have been encouraging. Biotechnology companies such as Vical and PowderMed are testing proto- type bird flu DNA vaccines.

Which Strain of Flu Virus should be Targeted for Vaccine Development?

With its genetic information composed of ribonucleic acid (RNA), the influenza virus is a constantly moving target by evolving very rapidly owing to its high mutating capacity, e.g. through random mutation. Genetic reas- sortment is a phenomenon involving the exchange of one or more of the eight genomic segments of a bird flu strain with the counterparts of a human flu strain when both viruses infect the same cell. The hybrid strain may acquire genes from both the bird and human viruses that encode proteins to which humans have no immunity, as well as gain the characteristics of heightened pathogenicity and human-to-human spread. Recombination is another mechanism of viral evolution whereby smaller genetic portions of a bird flu strain and another flu strain may be exchanged. Pigs are thought to be efficient "mixing vessels" for such genetic exchanges to occur.[16]

It is believed that the culprit pathogen that caused the flu pandemic responsible for decimating millions at the end of World War I was not a human flu virus but was a bird flu virus that had acquired the ability for human-to-human transmission.[17] Scientists are concerned that the H5N1 virus may eventually undergo random mutation or combination with a human flu virus to attain an enhanced competence for person-to-person spread. The increased genetic diversity of H5N1, and its existence in geo- graphically dispersed places in Asia, Europe and Africa may be a harbinger of rapid human transmission leading to a worldwide pandemic and possi- bly millions of fatalities. A worrying trend is that the bird flu strains that are presently circulating globally have mutated since originating from Asia in 2003. These strains possess specific mutations that render them significantly different from the initial outbreak strains.[18]

At this point in time, no definitive pandemic bird flu vaccine is avail- able, but prototype vaccines against H5N1 have been prepared or are being developed. For example, after H5N1 avian influenza first appeared in Hong Kong in 1997, a human vaccine was prepared but never fully developed or used. Drug companies are also attempting to generate a safe vaccine by manipulating a sample strain isolated from victims of the illness (e.g. a 2004 Vietnam strain). Some countries are even planning to stockpile such vaccines for future use. Even though the protective efficacy of these vaccines against pandemic flu would be dependent on how radically the virus evolves, they may protect against a variety of different but related strains. Although there is no guarantee that such vaccines will offer adequate protection against any human pandemic strain that ultimately emerges, it would be better to be ready with a vaccine at least related to the strain now circulating worldwide than to have none at all.

Currently, no one can forecast the exact influenza virus strain capable of causing a pandemic, and no one knows precisely what strain (which may not be H5N1) should be selected for developing a vaccine. However, should a pandemic be declared, and once the causative viral strain responsible for the pandemic is identified by WHO, the process of developing and testing a vaccine may take six months or more.

Can Sufficient Quantities of Flu Vaccines be Produced in Time when a Pandemic Strikes?

The existence of a vaccine in itself would be insufficient to avert a pandemic. Health experts highlight a chronic mismatch between public health requirements and the control of production of vaccines and drugs by private industry. One of the major scientific and logistic bottlenecks is to generate adequate supplies of vaccines to secure widespread protection.

For many years, the critical and unresolved problem is vaccine production capability. The capricious production process is an enormous challenge because it requires cultivation in fertilized chicken eggs. Vaccine production can take months, and is dependent on the number of eggs that farmers can supply to manufacturers. Furthermore, H5N1 flu vaccine production is likely to be even more challenging, since this strain is lethal in chickens. Another issue is the relatively high quantity of experimental vaccine required to induce immunity to the bird flu virus, i.e. about six times the normal dose necessary to protect against seasonal influenza. With some scientists proposing two separate injections of vaccine to ensure adequate protection, this will exert further pressure on production.

Currently, the global flu vaccine capacity is estimated to be 350 to 450 million doses annually, i.e. a mere fraction of the requirements for full coverage of the world's population. Even a developed country with an excellent health care infrastructure like the US faces a serious shortage of vaccines, having only enough doses for less than 2% of its population. In October 2005, President George Bush met the top executives of several large vaccine manufacturers including Sanofi-Aventis, GlaxoSmithKline and Merck, urging them to do their utmost to accelerate flu vaccine production. An imperative and important focus is to scale up and sustain short-term as well as long-term manufacturing capacity for influenza vaccines to meet the expected tremendous demand for pandemic vaccines. In March 2006, the US Food and Drug Administration announced proposals to establish an accelerated approval mechanism for authorizing production of new and seasonal flu vaccines.

It is extremely unlikely that sufficiently large quantities of human vaccines can be produced prior to the beginning of the flu pandemic. In reality, six months or more would be needed to produce enough vaccines to confront an influenza pandemic. Judging from the experience of previous pandemics, Dr. Anthony Fauci of the US National Institute of Allergy and Infectious Diseases predicts that a flu pandemic may begin with an initial wave of cases in one area. The epidemic may not reach global proportions until the following year, thus allowing vaccine manufacturers more time to respond. In particular scenarios, some researchers suggest that tactically deploying antiviral drugs may contain or even eliminate an outbreak of human influenza, and drastically reduce the number of subsequent deaths. Such a strategy may delay the spread of infection by a month or more, thus providing a respite while awaiting the availability of a vaccine.[19,20]

How Effective will Pandemic Bird Flu Vaccines be?

In 2005, Sanofi-Aventis, a French pharmaceutical company, announced successful results from preliminary trials of a vaccine against the fatal H5N1 bird flu strain. The "pre-pandemic" vaccine was developed in advance of the possible mutation of the H5N1 virus into a lethal pandemic version. Preliminary results demonstrated that the vaccine is safe, well-tolerated, and induces a dose-response curve that is expected to confer protective immunity. Immunization stimulated a strong immune response potent enough to neutralize the H5N1 strain. These promising results were based on a study involving healthy adult volunteers under 65 years of age who were injected with two doses of the vaccine. Tests to determine whether it will protect those most vulnerable to flu (i.e. children, elderly and people with chronic diseases) are expected to be completed in 2006. Despite this preliminary optimism, it is unclear whether a vaccine now being produced would be effective against an emergent pandemic strain. Moreover, some scientists advise caution on the overall effectiveness of this vaccine since vaccinees cannot be directly challenged with the deadly bird flu virus to confirm protection due to ethical reasons.

In addition, GlaxoSmithKline is developing a vaccine against the H5N1 bird flu strain which will be subjected to clinical trials in 2006. The Chinese Center for Disease Control and Prevention together with Sinovac Biotech company in Beijing have also jointly developed a prototype bird flu vaccine, and have commenced two-phase human trials in 2005. Other researchers are attempting to genetically engineer bird flu vaccines that can induce antibodies and elicit cell-mediated immunity against H5N1, and that can protect against viral mutants.

A good vaccine would be one that is a good match for the pandemic virus, decreases viral loads, and shows standardized potency such that the majority of vaccinees (e.g. three quarters) would be well-protected, while the rest suffer only from milder illness. On the other hand, bad vaccines mask signs of illness, but allow asymptomatic transmission as virus replication, shedding and evolution persists. Another undesirable consequence of flu immunization would be the emergence of vaccine-induced virus escape mutants.

Who should be Vaccinated Against Pandemic Flu?

In the event of a flu pandemic crisis, WHO has warned of the limited availability of vaccines and antiviral drugs. Scientists propose the implementation of international programs to distribute sufficient vaccines to people in less developed nations such as Cambodia, Indonesia and Vietnam, where most of the bird flu deaths have occurred and where a pandemic is likely to originate. If richer nations are willing to donate and assure supplies of vaccines and antiviral drugs, this would encourage poorer countries to cooperate on surveillance and preparedness.

Should a flu pandemic ignite, it is expected to strike in two waves. In any ideal national immunization plan, the entire population should be vaccinated before the second wave to significantly decrease the number of human infections and deaths. This strategy will necessitate the timely establishment of community vaccination centers, prompt and sufficient supplies of pandemic vaccine once it is available about six months following identification of the causative virus strain.

In the case of a pandemic with a scenario of severely limited vaccine stockpiles, tough decisions need to be made on who should get vaccinated. In view of such restrictions, priority may have to be given to high-risk groups such as health care personnel (e.g. doctors and nurses), poultry farmers, veterinary and laboratory workers in afflicted regions to prevent them from getting infected by their patients or animals.

Should Poultry and Other Animals be Vaccinated Against Bird Flu?

Although culling of infected poultry and other farm animals is the recommended method of stemming the spread of bird flu, poultry vaccination is practised as an experimental control measure in some parts of China, Indonesia and Thailand. This is a controversial and complex issue that has yet to be resolved.

Proponents of large-scale vaccination of poultry and other birds suggest that this could create a barrier to curb the spread of bird flu virus to humans. However, some scientists argue that vaccination would be unable to restrain the rapid and relentless deaths that ensue once bird flu infects a flock of farm birds. Furthermore, in Southeast Asia and other developing regions, control efforts are frequently hindered by ineffective and even fake agricultural vaccines. Farmers also worry that consumers may be unwilling to eat meat from vaccinated birds.

In response to several H5N1 outbreaks in birds in China in late 2005, veterinary officials pledged to immunize all 14 billion poultry in the country. But doubts are being expressed on whether the widespread vaccination of poultry can curtail human infections. Prior to the vaccination campaign, great numbers of infected birds died. By indicating the presence of the virus, this early warning sign could facilitate the early detection of human cases. However, after poultry vaccination, humans could get infected even though the birds appeared well, indicating that the virus in the animals has mutated. Some animals can thus act as asymptomatic carriers and can potentially excrete the virus. Although vaccines can provide some protection in animals, more research needs to be conducted on the effectiveness of poultry vaccination, and its impact on animal and human health as well as on surveillance systems.

What are the Economic and Cost-Benefit Issues of a Pandemic Flu Vaccine?

While there were less than 800 deaths attributed to the severe acute respiratory syndrome (SARS) outbreak throughout the world in 2003, its economic cost has been estimated at US$30 billion. In comparison, the economic, social and political consequences of a human influenza pandemic are expected to be calamitous, and no government can afford to be caught unprepared. Among Americans in the US, it is predicted that more than two million will die and nearly nine million will be hospitalized, with costs exceeding US$450 billion. The Lowy Institute for International Policy in Australia has estimated 140 million deaths worldwide and losses in global economic output amounting to US$4.4 trillion in a worst-case scenario.

In contrast, the costs of purchasing more antiviral drugs, investing in vaccines, forging national and international preparedness plans would be relatively much lower, but such measures may be critical. In November 2005, US President George Bush requested for US$7.1 billion in emergency funding for the campaign against a possible bird flu-related pandemic. The amount includes US$1 billion to stockpile more antiviral drugs, US$1.2 billion to produce approximately 20 million doses of a H5N1 vaccine, and US$2.8 billion to accelerate new influenza vaccine technology. In January 2006, international donors at a conference in Beijing pledged US$1.9 billion to support a global fund to fight bird flu. One of the priorities is to increase cooperation in global research and development of effective and safe animal and human vaccines, and to promote affordable access for all.

The reasons for the reluctance of pharmaceutical companies to produce more flu vaccines are varied. Flu vaccines are not very profitable as new batches must be produced for each winter season, with manufacturers often discarding millions of unused doses. Economic feasibility and intellectual property issues constitute a major hurdle, including expensive production costs and patent rights surrounding new techniques. In many countries including Singapore, a major weakness is the lack of production facilities for manufacturing vaccines in the event of an influenza pandemic. Vaccine manufacturers may not consider it a financially viable proposition to invest millions of dollars to build vaccine factories, if they are unable to recover their investments should a pandemic not materialize.

Without subjecting new vaccines to stringent safety trials before commercialization, drug companies also fear hefty lawsuits if healthy people suffer adverse effects following immunization. President Bush has also asked Congress to enact legislation to reduce this potentially considerable liability for influenza vaccine makers.

Will there be a Need to Generate New Bird Flu Vaccines in Future?

Scientists in the Netherlands and Sweden have reported that wild ducks, particularly mallards, harbor more than six avian influenza virus strains, and may be useful for monitoring and prediction of outbreaks. Their study supported the classical notion that wild birds carry the relatively avirulent viruses that ultimately mutate into highly pathogenic avian influenza strains. These researchers propose that influenza A surveillance in wild birds may serve as an early warning system since highly pathogenic avian influenza outbreaks in poultry arise from low pathogenic avian influenza viruses present in waterfowl. A stockpile of potential vaccines against future outbreaks in both animals and humans may also be accumulated by sampling influenza strains from these birds.[21]

In another study, samples taken from more than 13,000 migratory birds in Hong Kong and Jiangxi, China, during three winter seasons revealed that the H5N1 virus exists in healthy birds. This study also discovered that the lethal virus has evolved into four distinct gene families, implying that a single bird flu vaccine would not be able to control a human flu pandemic sparked by H5N1.[22]

A valuable lesson from these studies is that vaccines will probably need to be continuously and rapidly developed in future to battle potentially new lethal mutant variants of the bird flu virus.

Disclaimer

The author declares that he has not directly received any sponsorship in the form of research support, grants, honoraria, travel expenses or lecture fees from the commercial companies mentioned in this chapter.

References

1. Kawaoka Y (ed.) *Influenza Virology: Current Topics.* Caister Academic Press, Linton, UK, 2006.
2. Taubenberger JK, Morens DM. 1918 Influenza: the mother of all pandemics. *Emerg Infect Dis* 2006;12:15–22.
3. Buxton Bridges C, Katz JM, Seto WH, Chan PK, Tsang D, Ho W, Mak KH, Lim W, Tam JS, Clarke M, Williams SG, Mounts AW, Bresee JS, Conn LA, Rowe T, Hu-Primmer J, Abernathy RA, Lu X, Cox NJ, Fukuda K. Risk of influenza A (H5N1) infection among health care workers exposed to patients with influenza A (H5N1), Hong Kong. *J Infect Dis* 2000;181:344–348.
4. Fauci AS. Pandemic influenza threat and preparedness. *Emerg Infect Dis* 2006;12:73–77.
5. Lee VJ, Phua KH, Chen MI, Chow A, Ma S, Goh KT, Leo YS. Economics of neuraminidase inhibitor stockpiling for pandemic influenza, Singapore. *Emerg Infect Dis* 2006;12:95–102.
6. World Health Organization Writing Group. Non-pharmaceutical interventions for pandemic influenza: international measures. *Emerg Infect Dis* 2006; 12:81–87.
7. World Health Organization Writing Group. Non-pharmaceutical interventions for pandemic influenza: national and community measures. *Emerg Infect Dis* 2006;12:88–94.
8. de Jong MD, Tran TT, Truong HK, Vo MH, Smith GJ, Nguyen VC, Bach VC, Phan TQ, Do QH, Guan Y, Peiris JS, Tran TH, Farrar J. Oseltamivir resistance during treatment of influenza A (H5N1) infection. *New Engl J Med* 2005;353:2667–2672.

9. Luke CJ, Subbarao K. Vaccines for pandemic influenza. *Emerg Infect Dis* 2006;12:66–72.

10. Monto AS. Vaccines and antiviral drugs in pandemic preparedness. *Emerg Infect Dis* 2006;12:55–60.

11. Webby RJ, Perez DR, Coleman JS, Guan Y, Knight JH, Govorkova EA, McClain-Moss LR, Peiris JS, Rehg JE, Tuomanen EI, Webster RG. Responsiveness to a pandemic alert: use of reverse genetics for rapid development of influenza vaccines. *Lancet* 2004;363:1099–1103.

12. Lipatov AS, Webby RJ, Govorkova EA, Krauss S, Webster RG. Efficacy of H5 influenza vaccines produced by reverse genetics in a lethal mouse model. *J Infect Dis* 2005;191:1216–1220.

13. Palese P. Making better influenza virus vaccines? *Emerg Infect Dis* 2006;12:61–65.

14. Oxford JS, Manuguerra C, Kistner O, Linde A, Kunze M, Lange W, Schweiger B, Spala G, Rebelo de Andrade H, Perez Brena PR, Beytout J, Brydak L, Caraffa de Stefano D, Hungnes O, Kyncl J, Montomoli E, Gil de Miguel A, Vranckx R, Osterhaus A. A new European perspective of influenza pandemic planning with a particular focus on the role of mammalian cell culture vaccines. *Vaccine* 2005;23:5440–5449.

15. Epstein SL, Tumpey TM, Misplon JA, Lo CY, Cooper LA, Subbarao K, Renshaw M, Sambhara S, Katz JM. DNA vaccine expressing conserved influenza virus proteins protective against H5N1 challenge infection in mice. *Emerg Infect Dis* 2002;8:796–801.

16. Hollenbeck JE. An avian connection as a catalyst to the 1918–1919 influenza pandemic. *Int J Med Sci* 2005;2:87–90.

17. Taubenberger JK, Reid AH, Lourens RM, Wang R, Jin G, Fanning TG. Characterization of the 1918 influenza virus polymerase genes. *Nature* 2005;437:889–893.

18. Normile D. Infectious diseases: genetic analyses suggest bird flu virus is evolving. *Science* 2005;308:1234–1235.

19. Ferguson NM, Cummings DA, Cauchemez S, Fraser C, Riley S, Meeyai A, Iamsirithaworn S, Burke DS. Strategies for containing an emerging influenza pandemic in Southeast Asia. *Nature* 2005;437:209–214.

20. Longini IM, Nizam A, Xu S, Ungchusak K, Hanshaoworakul W, Cummings DA, Halloran ME. Containing pandemic influenza at the source. *Science* 2005;309:1083–1087.

21. Munster VJ, Wallensten A, Baas C, Rimmelzwaan GF, Schutten M, Olsen B, Osterhaus AD, Fouchier RA. Mallards and highly pathogenic avian influenza ancestral viruses, northern Europe. *Emerg Infect Dis* 2005;11:1545–1551.

22. Chen H, Smith GJ, Li KS, Wang J, Fan XH, Rayner JM, Vijaykrishna D, Zhang JX, Zhang LJ, Guo CT, Cheung CL, Xu KM, Duan L, Huang K, Qin K, Leung YH, Wu WL, Lu HR, Chen Y, Xia NS, Naipospos TS, Yuen KY, Hassan SS, Bahri S, Nguyen TD, Webster RG, Peiris JS, Guan Y. Establishment of multiple sublineages of H5N1 influenza virus in Asia: implications for pandemic control. *Proc Nat Acad Sci USA* 2006;103:2845–2850.

Some Related World Wide Web Sites

www.birdflu-vaccine.net
www.cdc.gov
www.flu.gov.sg
www.pandemicflu.gov
www.promedmail.org
www.who.int

13

Estimating Reduction in Hospitalizations Resulting from Different Levels of Antiviral Use During an Influenza Pandemic

Raymond Gani

The H5N1 strain of highly pathogenic avian influenza has spread from its origins in China to across Asia and into Europe despite efforts to control and contain its spread.[1] As a consequence, more people are likely to be exposed to the virus, which may increase the possibility of the emergence of a pandemic strain from this zoonotic strain. Should a pandemic strain emerge, national governments will be called upon to act to limit mortality and morbidity within their borders. A number of options will be available to reduce the severity of a pandemic, including both therapeutic and non-therapeutic interventions. Non-therapeutic options tend to focus on behavioral changes aimed at reducing transmission such as the closure of schools and discouraging mass gatherings, such as concerts and football matches, and advice on hygiene, hand washing and self-quarantine of infectious individuals.[2] Whilst these interventions may reduce transmission, it is not clear how effective they will be or how they will impact on total rates of mortality and morbidity.

Therapeutic options currently available for seasonal influenza are thought likely to be effective against pandemic influenza. Routine vaccination targeted at high-risk groups is common in many countries and leads to reduced morbidity and mortality. A trivalent vaccine is used each year in the UK and elsewhere to protect individuals against the currently prevalent circulating strains, usually two strains of influenza A and one strain of influenza B. During a pandemic, vaccine production capacity could be redirected to produce a single monovalent vaccine effective only against the circulating pandemic strain. However, a vaccine cannot begin to be produced before a pandemic begins, as the pandemic strain is required to produce an effective vaccine. Although alternative vaccine strategies are being considered and developed, it may take up a number of months before mass production of a pandemic vaccine begins, by which time the more severe aspects of a pandemic may be over.[3,4]

An alternative therapeutic option is the use of influenza antiviral drugs, which are effective against all strains of influenza A. Two groups of antiviral drugs are currently available for both treatment and prophylaxis of influenza. These are the adamantanes (amantadine and rimantadine) and neuraminidase inhibitors (oseltamivir and zanamivir). The adamantanes may be effective against pandemic strains but there are concerns over adverse reactions, especially in the elderly who most often constitute those most at risk of severe complications from influenza. There are also concerns over the development of resistance to these drugs. In the UK, amantadine is currently licensed for prophylaxis and treatment of influenza A but not recommended, due to side effects and the high likelihood of resistance.[5] The neuraminidase inhibitors (NIs) were developed more recently and have been shown to reduce the period of symptomatic illness from both influenza A and B viruses[6] and are licensed in the UK for both treatment and prophylaxis. Currently oseltamivir and zanamivir are both recommended for use during periods when influenza is known to be circulating in the UK for the treatment of at-risk adults who are able to commence treatment within 48 hours of the onset of symptoms. Additionally, oseltamivir is recommended for the treatment of at-risk children over the age of 12 months old. Oseltamivir is further recommended for post-exposure prophylaxis of at-risk adults and adolescents able to commence treatment within the 48 hours of close contact with an individual suffering from influenza-like illness. It is also recommended as prophylaxis for residents of care establishments for use post-exposure once influenza has been diagnosed in the establishment.[5] There are very few contra-indications to NIs and the majority have minimal side effects, though there are ongoing concerns regarding bronchospasm following the use of zanamivir. The development of antiviral resistance has been reported for NIs[7] though current evidence suggests that resistant strains are pathogenically enfeebled.[8] However, whilst the NIs are currently under licence and much more expensive than the adamantanes, the use of NIs for prophylaxis and treatment of influenza is an attractive option in the event of a pandemic as they will inevitably impact on the burden of disease.

A number of ways in which NIs could be used during a pandemic have been considered. The first is the prophylactic use of antivirals, where individuals exposed to infectious individuals are given the drug without it being known whether or not they have been infected. This will either prevent them developing symptoms if they were infected, or it will prevent them being infected if they are exposed in the future whilst still on prophylaxis. This option may delay spread and even contain small outbreaks, and is considered an option in the early stages of a pandemic in the index country. Here, in conjunction with other fairly stringent interventions, an attempt could possibly be made to contain the pandemic strain at source by preventing further spread within the index country and to other connected countries.[9,10] This option would require relatively large numbers of courses of antivirals but could result in the pandemic being stopped in its early stages. However, this strategy of prophylaxis is unlikely to be effective once international spread has begun, as non-index countries would be expected to have multiple importations. This would mean that the process of containment would need to be applied repeatedly in these countries and would lead to a rapid depletion of antiviral stockpiles. As many of those receiving prophylaxis will not have been infected, and therefore will not be immune, once the stockpile is depleted it is likely that the epidemic would reignite. Therefore, once international dissemination of the virus has occurred, this strategy is unlikely to contain a pandemic but it may delay more widespread incidence within a country for a short period of time.[11] This may only be of benefit if the current pandemic wave can be delayed sufficiently to provide enough time for a vaccine to be manufactured.

An alternative strategy for the use of NIs is for the treatment of symptomatic cases. Studies on the treatment of seasonal influenza with NIs suggest that when treatment is administered within 48 hours of onset of symptoms, there is an estimated 50% reduction in the likelihood of complications. On the basis of this relatively limited data, it is being widely assumed that, on average during a pandemic, treatment will result in a 50% reduction in the probability of hospitalization and a 50% reduction in the probability of death. In addition, studies have shown an estimated 1.5 day reduction in the duration of symptoms.[6] This reduction in the symptomatic period may also reduce the infectious period leading to reduced transmissibility. If widespread treatment was possible, the resulting reduction in the transmission rate may be enough to reduce the overall average transmission rate, leading to fewer cases overall. Unlike with prophylaxis, those treated will develop an immune response to the virus because they were infected, which means that they are unlikely to be re-infected by the same virus. Even if the virus mutates sufficiently so that are re-infected, they may retain partial immunity leading to less severe symptoms. It is for these reasons that many countries are considering buying, or have already bought, large numbers of NI treatment courses to stockpile for use during a pandemic.

Once the decision has been taken to stockpile NIs for treatment, the next question is how many courses to order and of which type. Of the two types available, oseltamivir is most commonly being stockpiled. Whilst the price and effectiveness of the two types of NIs are similar, their method of administration differs. Oseltamivir is taken orally but zanamivir needs to be inhaled, making oseltamivir easier to administer.

The decision on the size of the stockpile will probably depend on a number of factors such as the cost of the antivirals, the likelihood of a pandemic and competing health care demands. However, the starting point of any assessment will be to estimate what could be achieved with a stockpile of different sizes. Estimating this is fraught with problems, most pertinently we do not know what the characteristics of the next pandemic will be. The guide that we have however is our experience of previous pandemics and seasonal influenza A epidemics. In this chapter we will show that by using mathematical models, we can reproduce some of the salient features of previous pandemics, and then combined with contemporary data, assess what might happen today if the previous pandemic strains were to have occurred today. Once we are able to reproduce key features of previous pandemics with a model, we can then introduce intervention strategies into the model to determine their potential outcome. In this case the intervention that we assess is the treatment of symptomatic cases. We simulate a variety of different scenarios, for different sized stockpiles, to enable us to see not only how many cases might be prevented but also what the impact might be of running out of drugs. Using the model, we assess the outcome of the pandemic in terms of the number of hospital admissions or deaths. We also look at how a range of different targeted treatment strategies can be used to optimize the use of different sized stockpiles.

The starting point is the construction of an infectious disease model. Here, this begins by defining the various states of illness that a person infected with pandemic influenza will experience. Whilst the symptoms and severity of the disease has varied across previous pandemics and during seasonal influenza epidemics, the key elements required for the purposes of the model have remained more constant. The progression of the disease in an individual following infection is for that person to initially experience an asymptomatic latent period, where the individual experiences no symptoms and is not infectious. This period is followed by an infectious period, where the individual is contagious but will experience a range of severity of symptoms, from remaining asymptomatic, and therefore experiencing no symptoms, to experiencing severe complications which may result in death. In order for a person to be infected, the individual is required to be susceptible and, at least at the start of the first wave of a pandemic, this is likely to include the entire population. Following the infectious period, an individual will become immune to re-infection with the same virus. Whilst re-infection may occur following mutation of the virus, this is unlikely to occur within the same pandemic wave. It is the rate of transition between these four states, susceptible, latent, infectious and recovered, that forms the basis of the model.[12] The remaining part of the model, in the absence of interventions, is the transmission rate.

The transmission rate is a key feature of epidemic models and is composed of two elements. The first is dependent on the disease and relates to virus shedding and the second is behavioral and relates to human contact patterns involving infectious persons. These two aspects impact significantly on how effective different epidemic control measures might be. For example, patients with pneumonic plague are highly infectious only during the later stages of their disease. However, at this point they are usually easily identified because of their severe symptoms and can be isolated, usually resulting in few secondary cases.[13] During the severe acute respiratory syndrome (SARS) outbreak, those infected were not highly infectious until they were ill enough to be hospitalized. This led initially to many cases occurring in hospital, but once this was realized, and precautions taken to prevent this route of transmission, the disease was controlled.[14] There are, however, a number of factors that make influenza particularly difficult to control. Infected individuals are often infectious prior to the onset of symptoms meaning that they may have infected many people before they themselves realize that they have been infected. Those infected that remain asymptomatic may also infect others without ever knowing they were infected. In addition to this, tracing contacts of cases is difficult due to the relatively short incubation period for influenza. By contrast, during the smallpox eradication, contact tracing was made relatively easy due to the incubation period being 10–12 days, which enabled contacts to be found, quarantined and vaccinated.[15] However, with pandemic flu, given the relatively short generation time and potentially large number of exposed contacts, contact tracing would only be feasible for pandemic flu in the very earliest stages.

The transmission rate is often expressed as the basic reproduction number which in epidemic models is often denoted as R_0.[16] This value combines the two elements described above and represents the average number of secondary cases per primary case in an entirely susceptible population. This reference to a susceptible population is important because as the epidemic moves through a population, the number of secondary cases per infectious person falls, because the proportion of the population susceptible is falling, and therefore an infectious person is less likely to meet and infect a susceptible person. The definition for the transmission rate in a population that is not entirely susceptible is called the effective reproduction number and often denoted R_e. It can be calculated as

$$R_e = R_0 \times s$$

where s is the proportion of the population that is susceptible. R_e will decrease throughout an epidemic as the number of susceptible people decreases. Therefore R_0 can be viewed as a relatively invariant parameter relating to a particular disease for a particular epidemic, whilst R_e defines the observed infection rate at anytime throughout the epidemic. We shall revisit the concepts of R_0 and R_e in more detail later in the chapter, but for now suffice to say that if the value of R_0 is greater than one, an epidemic will occur until the value of R_e becomes less than one, at which point the epidemic will begin to subside, and it is the value of R_e which public health planners often seek to affect in order to control epidemics.

The next stage in the construction of the model is to include the impact of interventions. The scenarios we are considering here are the targeted treatment of clinical cases within different age and risk groups. In addition, antivirals are not recommended for those under one year old so they will not be treated in the model. Therefore the model is adapted to ensure that under the different scenarios the appropriate age and risk groups receive treatment. Also, given that treatment may reduce symptoms and therefore infectiousness, the model accounts for a reduction in the infectious period of all individuals that are treated.

The final stage is to run the model for different scenarios and calculate the outputs. In this instance we will be calculating the number of cases, hospitalizations and deaths each week. The model provides the number of cases per week by summing the number of individuals that become clinical cases during each week over the course of the simulated pandemic. To calculate the number of hospitalizations or deaths per week, the model uses the probability of hospitalization or death applied to each clinical case, as well as changes in these probabilities if clinical cases receive treatment. The number of hospitalizations or deaths is summed throughout each week to get weekly totals. A schematic of the model is shown in Figure 1 and the model is defined mathematically in the Appendix.

Once the model has been constructed, it needs to be parameterized. The robustness of the parameters will determine the confidence that can be placed in the results and the range of outputs that can be generated. For most models, parameters may be measured directly through experiments, such as case control studies or sampling, and when this is not available, surrogate data may be used. Seasonal influenza is perhaps the best surrogate for pandemic influenza when specific pandemic data are lacking. There are a number of aspects of pandemic flu that appear to be fairly consistent with seasonal influenza. These include the latent period, which is on average

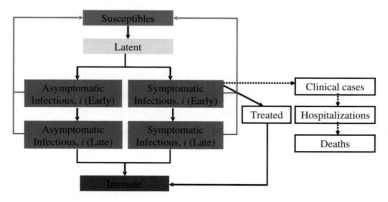

Figure 1: Schematic of the model used to determine the impact of antiviral treatment. Here the red boxes represent infectious states with red lines representing the route of infection of the susceptible group, given in green. Those in the susceptible group that are infected go on to become latent then infectious. Following the infectious period they enter the immune state, where they either recover or die. The clinical cases are calculated from those in the early symptomatic infectious state where they may or may not be treated. A fraction of these will become hospitalized or die, which may change due to treatment. As the clinical attack rates, and hospitalization and death rates, as well as treatment strategies may vary by risk and age, the model needs to be stratified by these, denoted i.

about two days, and the infectious period, which is on average of about four days long.[10] The effectiveness of treatment is expected to be similar between pandemic and seasonal strains, reducing symptoms on average by 1.5 days and reducing the probability of complications (by which we also assume hospitalization and death) by 50% as previously stated.

There are, however, a number of aspects of the previous pandemics that do vary considerably from seasonal influenza and indeed between pandemics. The previous three influenza pandemics that occurred during the 20th century had varying degrees of severity, with outcomes that have ranged from the high levels of mortality and morbidity observed during the 1918–19 "Spanish flu" pandemic, which resulted in an estimated 20–40 million deaths, to the much lower levels of mortality observed during the pandemics of 1957–58 and 1968–69, which resulted in approximately one million deaths each. Each of these pandemics also had different overall clinical attack rates, different age-specific attack rates, lasted for different periods of time and had different numbers of pandemic waves.[12,17]

The age-specific attack rate proportioned across different age groups for the main waves of the 1957 and 1968 pandemics in the UK, and for the three waves of the 1918 pandemic are shown in Table 1, which demonstrates not only the difference between pandemics, and between waves within pandemics, but also between seasonal influenza, which tends to exhibit the highest attack rates in both the very young and the elderly. Table 2 shows how a variety of other aspects have varied between pandemics. Hospitalization rates are given for the 1957 and 1968 pandemic but could not be ascertained for the 1918 pandemic. Overall clinical attack rates during the 1957, 1968 and the three waves of the 1918 pandemic are shown, and these vary considerably. Case fatality rates for the different waves of the 1918 pandemic are shown, which are considerably higher than those for the 1957 and 1968 pandemics, which were more comparable case fatality rates observed

Table 1: Reported age-specific clinical attack rates for the different scenarios.

Age class (years)	0–4	5–14	15–64	65+
1957 (Ref. 22)	26%	42%	22%	10%
1968 (Ref. 23)	16%	11%	49%	24%
1918 1st Wave (Ref. 18)	16%	32%	43%	9%
1918 2nd Wave (Ref. 18)	27%	31%	29%	14%
1918 3rd Wave (Ref. 18)	24%	22%	29%	24%

Table 2: Parameters required for scenario specific simulations. Reported values for 1957 from Anon. (1960),[22] for 1968 from Barker and Mullooly (1980),[24] and for 1918 from Anon. (1920).[18]

	1957	1968	1918 1st wave	1918 2nd wave	1918 3rd wave
Overall hospitalization rate per 100,000 of the population	188[a]	144[a]	–	–	–
Overall clinical attack rate	31%[a]	21%[c]	5%[c]	9%[c]	4%[c]
% Immune at start of wave	0%[d]	15%[c]	0%[d]	0%[d]	0%[d]
R_0	1.65[b]	2.2[b]	2.00[b]	1.55[b]	1.70[b]
Case fatality rate	–	–	0.70%[a]	3.25%[a]	2.70%[a]

[a]Reported values; [b]calculated by fitting the model to data; [c]calculated directly from data; [d]assumed values.

for seasonal influenza (data not shown). Values of the transmission rate, R_0, are also given in Table 2 and their derivation is described below.

A key aspect to the epidemic models is the transmission rate R_0 as its value will determine a number of key aspects of the pandemic wave. These include the duration of the epidemic, the size of the peak and the total number of cases. Intervention policies will affect not R_0 (as it is invariant across the pandemic wave) but R_e, the effective reproduction number. The scale to which R_e is affected will determine the effectiveness of intervention policy. Indeed, for other transmissible diseases, the level of recommended coverage during mass vaccination campaigns, C, is often determined by the value

$$C < 1 - 1/R_0.$$

More specifically, if the proportion protected can be reduced, by vaccination or some other means, to a fraction of the population of C, then the disease is unlikely to cause a widespread epidemic. For diseases such as measles or chickenpox, the R_0 values are in the range of 11–18 and 7–12, respectively and the recommended vaccination coverages of 90%–95% and 85%–90% for these diseases.[16] The effectiveness of alternative control strategies can also be assessed with reference to R_0. For example, for contact tracing and isolation to be successful on its own, the proportion of infected contacts that need to be found must be greater than the value of $1 - 1/R_0$. Towards the end of the smallpox eradication campaign, existing mass vaccination attempts were supplemented by targeting contacts of infectious cases for vaccination and quarantine. For smallpox, R_0 was of the order of 4–5 meaning that the proportion of contacts needing to be found had to be greater than 75%–80%.[15] This was helped by the relatively long incubation period and contributed to smallpox eventually being eradicated.

What both these control strategies are attempting to achieve is to reduce the number of secondary cases per infected person to less than one. During an unconstrained epidemic, in which there are no effective control options to reduce transmission, we see a number of different phases, each of which can be viewed in terms of changes to R_e. During the first phase, the value of R_e is close to R_0 and we observe near exponential growth, that is the rate of increase in cases is relatively constant and at its greatest. As more people are infected, the pool of susceptible individuals starts to become depleted and we begin to see reductions in R_e. Near the peak of the pandemic, $R_e = 1$ and the proportion of susceptible population depleted is approximately $1 - 1/R_0$. The proportion of the population susceptible continues to fall over the final phases of the epidemic, as does the R_e. The epidemic will not recrudesce unless the proportion susceptible increases, such as through new births or waning immunity, or if the virus mutates sufficiently that those previously immune through previous infection becoming susceptible once more.

Therefore, given the impact of R_0 on the dynamics of the disease it is necessary to estimate it before any assessment of intervention strategies can begin. We do this here by numerically fitting the model to national incidence data from previous pandemics. This is done by using the model defined above to produce simulations for each of the pandemics using the parameters given above and assuming no treatment strategies are used. A range of values for R_0 are used in the model and the value which minimizes the error measure between the observations and the model outputs gives the best estimate of R_0 and is the value used subsequently in the further simulations. These values are given in Table 2. The fit of the model to the data for the different pandemics is shown in Figure 2.[12] The only remaining parameter for the model is the age- and risk-specific hospitalization rates. Given that data on these are not available for previous pandemics, the relative rates were derived from seasonal influenza (see Table 3) and then distributed across age and risk groups so that they aggregated to the observed rates from previous pandemics.[12] Whilst during seasonal flu, the elderly are worst affected, during a pandemic the attack rate in this group is lower. By using the attack rates from Table 1 and the hospitalization rates from Table 3 sequentially, this effect is included in the model and means that compared to a pandemic, the morbidity in this group is relatively lower than during seasonal flu. Overall hospitalization rates were only available for the 1957 and 1968 pandemics, so was not possible to assess hospitalization rates for the 1918 pandemic. However, given that mortality rates were available for 1918, an assessment on the impact of treatment on deaths was made.

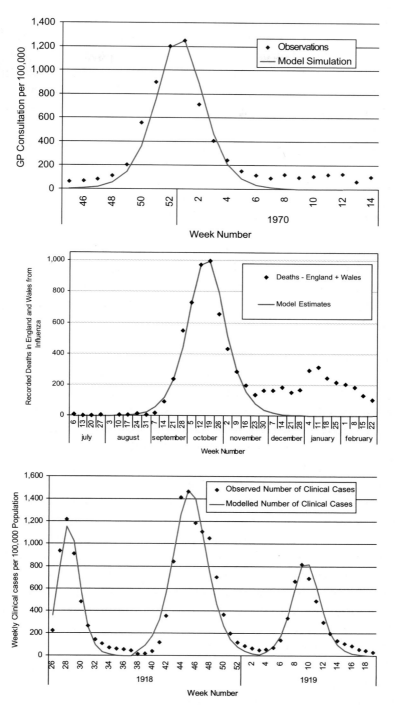

Figure 2: Model fitted to national pandemic influenza data from the main wave during winter 1969–70 of the 1968 Hong Kong flu pandemic (top), the main first wave of the 1957 Asian flu pandemic and the three waves of the 1918 Spanish flu pandemic.

Table 3: Relative hospitalization rates for clinical cases for different age and risk groups.[12]

Age (years)	Hospitalization rates per 100,000	
	High risk	Low risk
0–4	3,562	509
5–14	274	39
15–64	873	125
65–74	4,235	605
≤ 75	8,797	1,257

The model is now parameterized and ready to be used to produce simulations for a number of different treatment strategies. Given the variation in the parameters from the different pandemics, and the differences in the data available for the different pandemics, it was decided to simulate the three pandemics separately rather than produce a generic set of parameters from across previous pandemics. This would then be able to be used to indicate the variation in what might have been done given a pandemic today which had the same features as one from the past with different sized stockpiles and treatment strategies. The current parameterization of the model for the different pandemics will not necessarily reproduce the next or a future pandemic. This approach is intended purely to give policy makers an idea of what might be expected. If a pandemic were to occur, any model would have to be re-parameterized with data specifically relating to the current pandemic and re-run at the earliest opportunity. One of the most difficult aspects of this re-parameterization will be the estimation of R_0, which will require the use of other real-time models beyond the scope of this chapter.

We now consider four intervention strategies related to the targeted treatment of clinical cases, and measure its effectiveness by estimating the expected number of people requiring hospitalization and the number of deaths. The four treatment groups were defined based on potential treatment options. One treatment group to be targeted for treatment are those in at-risk groups as defined for seasonal influenza as this is a strategy that might be employed where antiviral treatment is limited. A second group are those over the age of 65 years and those under the age of 12 as they could be easily identified and also include the majority of those at risk from seasonal influenza. A third group are those of working age, a strategy that might be considered in order to maintain economic resilience. A fourth option examined was to treat all clinical cases. The simulations would model different stockpile sizes by varying the number of treatments that could be administered. For each of the four treatment strategies, NI treatments would be administered until the stockpile was exhausted. Treatments were assumed to be administered within 48 hours of onset of symptoms, to simulate the best outcome that could be achieved under each particular strategy.

The effect on hospitalization rates is shown in Figure 3 for the 1957 and 1968 pandemics. For each of the sets of simulations, there is a near

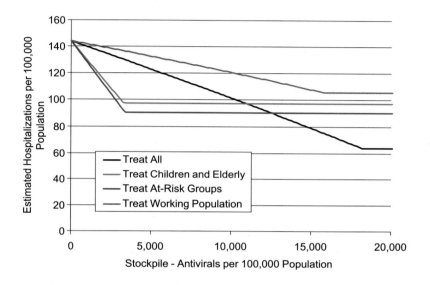

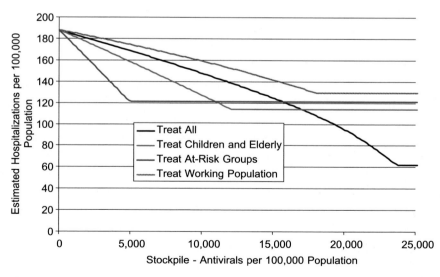

Figure 3: Estimated hospital admission rates for different treatment strategies at different stockpile sizes when the model is parameterized for the 1968 (left) and 1957 (right) pandemics. *Source:* Modified from Figures 3 and 4 of Ref. 12.

linear decrease in the hospitalization rates until a point at which the impact becomes constant, shown in the graphs as the horizontal part of the curves. At this point, the stockpile is sufficient in size to treat all clinical cases in the proposed group and therefore, once they are all treated any additional increase in stockpile size will not lead to any additional benefit. Whilst it may be argued that at this point, different groups would begin to be treated, it should be noted that these are the hospitalization rates across the entire pandemic and calculated at its end. Therefore the excess stockpile would not be realized until late into the pandemic, by which time it would be largely too late to change strategies. Another feature is that for some of the scenarios there is an apparently linear decrease in hospitalization rate with increasing stockpile size, whilst for others the hospitalization rate decreases by an increasing rate as stockpile size increases. This is due to the impact on the transmission rate caused by the reduction in the infectious period assumed for antiviral treatment. The result of this is that as treatment increases, the impact on transmission increases and the total number of clinical cases falls. This in turn leads to fewer hospitalizations.

The impact of these different strategies varies across the two pandemics due to key differences in the parameterization (Tables 1 and 2). The overall hospitalization rate is higher for the simulations using the data from 1957 (Table 2), which is therefore reflected in the higher rates in Figure 3. The stockpile size required to treat all cases as a proportion of the population, is generally larger for the 1957 pandemic due to the higher overall clinical attack rate compared to 1968 (Table 2). There are qualitative differences between the relative effectiveness of the different strategies across the two pandemics, which are mainly due to differences in the age-specific attack rates that are given in Table 1. Of the four strategies, under any stockpile size, treating only the working population is the least effective strategy in reducing the hospitalization rate. This requires not only a large number of treatments as this group is large, but is also badly targeted as this group is effectively the least likely to develop complications and go to hospital. Treating all clinical cases is the best strategy for larger stockpiles, greater than around 11,000 treatment courses per 100,000 population for the 1968 pandemic and around 15,000 per 100,000 population for the 1957 pandemic. Treating all cases has the additional benefit using the 1957 data of reducing the average transmission rate thereby increasing the rate of decrease in the expected hospitalization rate as stockpile size is increased. Of the remaining two strategies considered, their impacts vary across the two pandemic. Using the 1968 data, they are roughly equivalent in their impact at all stockpile sizes, though the treatment of at-risk groups is slightly better. Using the

1957 data, the treatment of at-risk groups is much better to stockpile sizes of around 11,000 per 100,000, thereafter treatment of children and the elderly becomes more effective, followed by the treatment of all cases for the largest stockpiles (>18,000 per 100,000).

An illustration of what the simulated epidemic curves look like for the 1968 and 1957 pandemics is shown in Figure 4 for a selection of scenarios. When scenarios where there is no treatment are compared to scenarios where there is a stockpile sufficiently large to treat all clinical cases, the curves for the latter are flatter and broader and the resulting number of cases is lower. This is due to the effect of treatment on the transmission rate, which is reduced due to the shorting of the infectious period in treated individuals. For the scenario when all cases are treated but the stockpile size only covers 10% of the population, the epidemic initially follows the curve generated with the larger stockpile, until it runs out. Here, the transmission rate is no longer reduced due to treatment, and what follows is a rapid rise in the transmission rate which produces a sharp peak during the middle of the pandemic wave. Across both pandemics, when there is enough antiviral to treat 10% of the population, there is more than enough antiviral to treat all clinical cases in the at-risk groups. However, in spite of only treating this group and having a surplus remaining at the end of the wave, this is the best strategy as it results in the least hospitalizations due to the effectiveness with which treatment is targeted. It is therefore worth bearing in mind that what may initially look like the most effective policy, such as a decision to treat all clinical cases, may by the end of the epidemic not necessarily be so.

Simulations were produced next using parameters from the three waves of the 1918 pandemic. An extensive overview of the 1918 pandemic both in the UK and internationally can be found in the 1920 report from the UK Ministry of Health,[18] and it is from here that the data to parameterize the model for the 1918 pandemic has mostly been derived. The characteristics for the 1918 pandemic differ substantially from the other two pandemics in a number of ways. The first is that three large and distinct waves were observed, a characteristic that was observed almost worldwide. The second major difference was the unusual age-specific attack rate, shown in Table 1, where the elderly and young were relatively spared compared with those in their teens, 20s and 30s, who experienced the highest attack rates. The third major difference was in the scale of morbidity and mortality. The first wave lasted about six weeks, occurred in June and July 1918 and was described at the time as not being unusual compared to other pandemics that had occurred in the 19th and early 20th centuries. It also appears to have shared many of the characteristics of the 1957 and 1968 pandemics, all being relatively severe

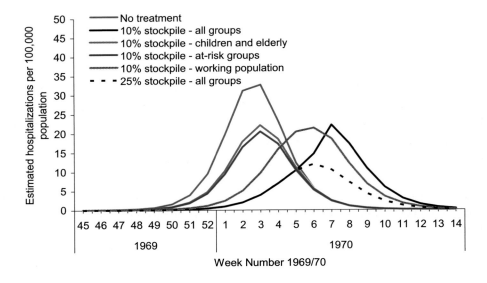

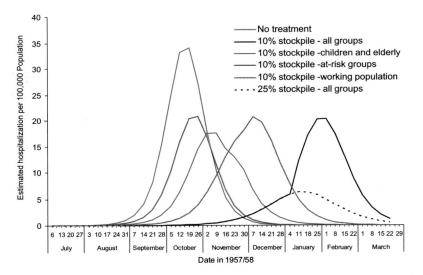

Figure 4: Selection of epidemic curves generated from the model parameterized from the 1968 (left) and the 1957 (right) pandemics. The red curves show no treatment, the dashed black curve shows all clinical cases treated, and the remaining curves are when there is a stockpile large enough to cover 10% of the population when all cases are treated (solid black curve), when only the working population is treated (purple curve), when only the young and elderly are treated (blue curve), and when only the at-risk groups are treated (green curve). *Source*: Modified from Figures 3 and 4 of Ref. 12.

forms of influenza. Although the age-specific attack rates were unusual, and morbidity and mortality rates were raised, they were not unusually high. Eight weeks after the first wave ceased, a second wave appeared in October and lasted for about 12 weeks. During this period over 100,000 deaths were attributed to this disease in England and Wales alone, with clinical features differing from typical influenza. Gross mortality rates in the UK were said to be at their highest level since the period of the Black Death in the 14th century. Whilst the majority of cases experienced typical, but severe forms of influenza, a large proportion also developed pulmonary complications. During the third wave, which began in February and lasted about eight weeks, mortality rates were high for influenza, but considerably lower than that observed during the second wave. It was noted that the third wave appeared to revert to being more like seasonal influenza, and attack rates were higher in the very young and elderly, compared to the first two waves.

Modeling with the 1918 pandemic data was therefore less straightforward than with the previous 1957 and 1968 data due to its multiple waves and the type of data available to parameterize the model. As less data was available for the 1918 pandemic, only the impact of two stockpile sizes was modeled and only on the expected number of deaths. The stockpile sizes modeled were one large enough to cover 10% of the population and another large enough to cover 20%. The approach taken to modeling the multiple waves was to fit the transmission model to each of the three waves separately to determine the R_0 for each wave. The parameters used were the age-specific attack rates (Table 1) and case fatality rates (Table 2) for each of the waves. The simulated outputs (Figure 5) are shown in terms of the total number of deaths per week for each of the two stockpile sizes compared with the scenario where there is no treatment. Based on the characteristics of the 1918 pandemic and in the absence of antiviral treatment but using contemporary UK demographic age profiles, the number of estimated deaths across the three waves would be approximately 0.5% of the total population. However, the actual number of cases would be less than those with assumptions based on the parameters of the 1957 or 1968 pandemics. Therefore the demand for treatment would be less. In this case a stockpile large enough to treat 20% of the population would be sufficient to treat all clinical cases across all three waves and reduce the number of deaths by about 53%. However, when the stockpile size is halved, the reduction in deaths is only 17%. This is because most of the stockpile is used up during the first wave which has a relatively low mortality rate and eventually becomes exhausted during the second wave, before most of the deaths have occurred.

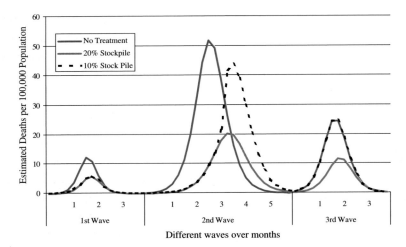

Figure 5: Expected number of deaths from the model parameterized from the three waves of the 1918 pandemic, when there is no treatment, a 20% antiviral stockpile, and a 10% antiviral stockpile. *Source*: From Figure 5 of Ref. 12.

The results illustrate that to considerably reduce excess hospitalizations and deaths during a pandemic through the widespread treatment of clinical cases, substantial stockpiles of NI are likely to be required. However, substantial reductions can also be achieved with smaller stockpiles if appropriately targeted to those at highest risk of complications. It will be vital to estimate the risk of hospitalization of different age and risk groups during the early stages of a pandemic in order optimize treatment strategies, especially if stockpiles are limited. The analyses demonstrate that during previous pandemics, antiviral coverage for 20%–25% of the population would likely have been sufficient to treat all clinical cases. If a future pandemic was to follow a similar type of behavior, with similar transmission and attack rates, then it would be expected that this size stockpile would be adequate for this purpose. However, in order for this strategy to be most effective, clinical cases must be treated within 48 hours of onset of symptoms and therefore treatment needs to be supported by good clinical judgement, diagnostic capability and clear strong public health messages, as well as distribution systems which will be effective even at the height of a pandemic.

Each pandemic is unique with its own characteristics, and optimal treatment strategies will vary between them. Whilst the results provided here are useful in helping to scope and quantify resource and planning requirements ahead of time, it is recognized that these results are of necessity based on limited data from previous pandemic and inter-pandemic influenza, expert opinion and clinical trials. Such assessments will need to be re-calculated in the earliest phases of a pandemic using real-time data to either confirm or update the assumptions used and ensure that model parameterization is appropriate for the new pandemic strain.

Appendix: Mathematical Model Used to Calculate Outputs

The model used was based on the theory of epidemic modeling given by Anderson and May (1991),[16] which has formed the basis of a number of models for both epidemic and pandemic influenza,[19–21] and implemented as the set of differential equations given below. Here, $\alpha = 1/LP = 0.5$, $\gamma = 1/PP = 0.4$, $\lambda = 1/IP = 2/3$ and $\beta = R_0/(PP+IP)$, LP is the latent period of two days, PP the initial part of the infectious period of 2.5 days, and IP is the second part of the infectious period of 1.5 days. S represents the total proportion susceptible, E the total proportion incubating, P_i the proportion from the total population in each age and risk group i within the first 2.5 days of their infectious period, I_i the proportion of total population in each age and risk group i within the final 1.5 days of their infectious period, and R the total proportion recovered and immune or dead. c_i is the proportion of infections resulting in clinical cases in each age and risk, and T_i proportion in each age and risk i receiving treatment. The average number of secondary cases per primary case when the population is entirely susceptible is represented by R_0 and the proportion of the population in each group i is given by N_i.

$$\frac{dS}{dt} = -\beta S \left(\sum_i P_i + I_i \right)$$

$$\frac{dE}{dt} = \beta S \left(\sum_i P_i + I_i \right) - \alpha E$$

$$\frac{dP_i}{dt} = \alpha N_i E - \gamma P_i$$

$$\frac{dI_i}{dt} = \gamma P_i (1 - c_i . T_i) - \lambda I_i$$

$$\frac{dR}{dt} = c \sum_i T_i + \lambda I_i.$$

The proportion of the population within each group being hospitalized each week, $H_i(t)$, can be calculated as

$$H_i(t) = \int_t^{t+7} \gamma P_i(t) c_i h_i (1 - \varepsilon T_i) dt$$

where ε the efficacy of antiviral treatment against hospitalization and h_i is the hospitalization rate for each group i. The proportion treated in each group each week can be given as $A(t)$ as

$$A_i(t) = \int_t^{t+7} \gamma P_i(t) c_i T_i dt$$

where t is time in days.

References

1. Webster RG, Peiris M, Chen H, Guan Y. H5N1 outbreaks and enzootic influenza. *Emerg Infect Dis* 2006;12(1):3–8.
2. WHO. *WHO Global Influenza Preparedness Plan*. World Health Organization, Geneva, 2005 (http://www.who.int/csr/resources/publications/influenza/GIP_2005_5Eweb.pdf).
3. Fedson DS. Pandemic influenza and the global vaccine supply. *Clin Infect Dis* 2003;36:1552–1561.
4. Webby RJ, Webster RG. Are we ready for pandemic influenza? *Science* 2003;302:1519–1522.
5. NICE. *Full Guidance on the Use of Zanamivir, Oseltamivir and Amantadine for the Treatment of Influenza*. National Institute for Clinical Excellence, UK, 2003 (http://www.nice.org.uk/pdf/58_Flu_fullguidance.pdf).
6. Stiver G. The treatment of influenza with antiviral drugs. *CMAJ* 2003;168:49–57.
7. Kiso M, Mitamura K, Sakai-Tagawa Y, Shiraishi K, Kawakami C, Kimura K, Hayden FG, Sugaya N, Kawaoka Y. Resistant influenza A viruses in children treated with oseltamivir: descriptive study. *Lancet* 2004;364:759–765.
8. McKimm-Breschkin J, Trivedi T, Hampson A, Hay A, Klimov A, Tashiro M, Hayden FG, Zambon M. Neuraminidase sequence analysis and susceptibilities of influenza virus clinical isolates to zanamivir and oseltamivir. *Antimicrob Agents Chemother* 2003;47:2264–2272.
9. Ferguson NM, Cummings DA, Cauchemez S, Fraser C, Riley S, Meeyai A, Iamsirithaworn S, Burke DS. Strategies for containing an emerging influenza pandemic in Southeast Asia. *Nature* 2005;437(7056):209–214.
10. Longini IM Jr, Nizam A, Xu S, Ungchusak K, Hanshaoworakul W, Cummings DA, Halloran ME. Containing pandemic influenza at the source. *Science* 2005;309(5737):1083–1087.
11. Longini IM Jr, Halloran ME, Nizam A, Yang Y. Containing pandemic influenza with antiviral agents. *Am J Epidemiol* 2004;159(7):623–633.
12. Gani R, Hughes H, Fleming D, Griffin T, Medlock J, Leach S. Potential impact of antiviral drug use during influenza pandemic. *Emerg Infect Dis* 2005;11(9):1355–1362.
13. Gani R, Leach S. Epidemiologic determinants for modeling pneumonic plague outbreaks. *Emerg Infect Dis* 2004;10(4):608–614.

14. Wenzel RP, Bearman G, Edmond MB. Lessons from severe acute respiratory syndrome (SARS): implications for infection control. *Arch Med Res* 2005;36(6):610–616.

15. Gani R, Leach S. Transmission potential of smallpox in contemporary populations. *Nature* 2001;414(6865):748–751.

16. Anderson RM, May RM. *Infectious Diseases of Humans: Dynamics and Control.* Oxford University Press, 1991.

17. Nguyen-Van-Tam JS, Hampson AW. The epidemiology and clinical impact of pandemic influenza. *Vaccine* 2003;21:1762–1768.

18. Anon. *Report on the Pandemic of Influenza 1918–19*, Reports on Public Health and Medical Subjects No. 4. Her Majesty's Stationary Office, London, 1920.

19. Rvachev LA, Longini IM. A mathematical model for the global spread of influenza. *Math Biosci* 1985;75:3–22.

20. Flahault A, Letrait S, Blin P, Hazout S, Menares J, Valleron AJ. Modelling the 1985 influenza epidemic in France. *Stat Med* 1988;7:1147–1155.

21. Flahault A, Deguen S, Valleron AJ. A mathematical model for the European spread of influenza. *Eur J Epidemiol* 1994;10:471–474.

22. Anon. *The Influenza Epidemic in England and Wales 1957–58*, Reports on Public Health and Medical Subjects No. 100. Her Majesty's Stationary Office, London, 1960.

23. Taylor MP. Influenza 1968–1970 incidence in general practice based on a population survey. *J R Coll Gen Pract* 1971;21:17–22.

24. Barker WH, Mullooly JP. Impact of epidemic type A influenza in a defined adult population. *Am J Epidemiol* 1980;112:798–811.

14

Hong Kong's Public Health Preparedness for Avian Influenza Pandemic[a] Under a Three-Tier Response System

Ronald M.-K. Lam and Pak-Yin Leung

Avian influenza is not new to Hong Kong. We first experienced an outbreak of the highly pathogenic H5N1 avian influenza among poultry in 1997, with 18 cases of human infection resulting in six deaths. A few sporadic cases occurred in later years, including three H5N1 outbreaks among poultry between 2001 to 2003 and two imported cases of H5N1 human infection detected in February 2003.

Investigations into the human cases incriminated contact with live poultry as the major route of infection and human-to-human transmission was found to be inefficient.[b] Appropriate control strategies, including

---

[a]An influenza pandemic is a global outbreak of disease that occurs when a new influenza virus appears or "re-emerges" in the human population against which the human has no immunity, spreads and causes disease worldwide.

[b]Efficient human-to-human transmission is defined as the ability of the virus to readily spread from person to person in the general population and cause multiple outbreaks of disease leading to epidemics.

depopulation of affected poultry,[c] control of import, wholesale and retail of poultry, reinforced surveillance and public health protection, etc. have enabled us to keep this enemy of avian influenza at bay. As a matter of fact, Hong Kong's effort in controlling the avian influenza outbreak in 1997 has been commended by international experts in having averted a possible impending pandemic.

Previous outbreaks and past incidents of human infection constantly remind us that avian influenza outbreaks in poultry populations pose significant threat to public health. The risk has become more imminent with waves of avian influenza springing up in different parts of the world in recent years.

Renewed and Rising Threats

Since January 2004, human infections of H5N1 avian influenza have been reported in Vietnam, Thailand, Cambodia, Indonesia, as well as in mainland China from July 2005. At the time of writing,[d] 141 cases (73 deaths) were reported to the World Health Organization (WHO) and the human infections were either preceded by, or occurring concomitantly with, large outbreaks of avian influenza among poultry. There is also increasing evidence that the H5N1 virus is spreading via the migratory birds westwards reaching as far as Europe and the host range has widened with infections detected in mammals such as tigers.

According to WHO, the H5N1 virus is now firmly entrenched in large parts of Asia and thus the risk that more human infection cases will occur will persist. Each new case will give the virus an additional opportunity to improve its transmissibility to humans and thus a higher potential to develop into a pandemic strain. The recent spread of the virus to poultry and wild birds in new areas further broadens opportunities for human cases to occur. While neither the timing nor the severity of the next pandemic can be predicted, the probability that a pandemic will occur has increased.

Ongoing Public Health Preparedness

The Hong Kong Special Administrative Region Government is committed to safeguarding the health of the community. Proactive preparation and

---

[c]In the avian influenza outbreak of 1997, over 1.6 million chickens and other poultry were slaughtered in all local chicken farms, poultry wholesale markets and retail outlets.
[d]Figures as of 29 December 2005.

planning for the prevention of influenza pandemic have been progressively strengthened after the challenge of the first avian influenza outbreak in 1997.

Removing the source of infection is a foremost objective of disease prevention. Hong Kong has geared up veterinary public health measures to guard against the occurrence of avian influenza outbreaks by targeting at poultry as reservoir for infection. They include vaccination of chickens; enforcement of tightened bio-security measures in local poultry farms; import control and antibody level testing on imported chickens; monitoring of dead and sick birds; segregation policy; market rest days for cleansing and disinfection; specific hygiene/disinfection requirements on wholesale markets and retail outlets, transport cages and vehicles, etc. In addition, poultry retailers will be required to surrender all live poultry for disposal on detection of even one dead bird with H5 virus isolated.

Efforts are also made to minimize health risk by *reducing contact between humans and live poultry* as far as possible since experience indicates that the principal mode of transmission of avian influenza virus from poultry to humans is through contact with infected poultry or their feces. To achieve this objective, since the year 2005, the maximum licence capacity of local poultry farms has been reduced, and a voluntary scheme has been introduced for licensed live poultry farmers, wholesalers and transporters to surrender their licences or tenancies, in return for *ex-gratia* payment, to cease operation permanently. Meanwhile, the government is considering central slaughtering of poultry as a long-term measure to separate humans from live poultry.

Ongoing human health protection functions are further enhanced with the setting up of a Centre for Health Protection (CHP) under the Department of Health on 1 June 2004. The CHP adopts a multidisciplinary and integrated approach, and maintains close working relationships with national, regional and local healthcare professionals and organizations for effective disease control. A scientific advisory structure comprising of a Board of Scientific Advisors and seven Scientific Committees has been set up. This collaborative arrangement has brought together knowledge and experience from across disciplines and institutes to formulate strategies and actions for communicable disease control.

Infection control (IC) is an effective way to prevent disease transmission. The government is building up its IC hardware by enhancing the facilities in hospitals[e] and institutions; by stockpiling personal protective equipment

---

[e]Over 1400 isolation beds are available in the Hospital Authority and a new infectious disease block in the Princess Margaret Hospital is scheduled for completion in 2006.

such as surgical masks, disinfectants and so forth, and is also advising the public to do so. With regard to IC software, policies and guidelines for different settings are developed and training of staff as well as caretakers in community and hospital settings arranged.

The magnitude of impact caused by a pandemic may overload any public health system. Hence, *surge capacity* is further enhanced by enlisting the support of the private sector, and volunteers are recruited from doctors, nurses, pharmacists, allied health professionals, social workers and non-governmental organizations to offer assistance.

Emergency Preparedness and Response

The universal basic assumption about avian influenza, should it evolve to a pandemic strain, is that the timing for this to occur is unpredictable, yet inevitable. No part of the globe will be spared and public health measures should therefore not only focus on merely prevention and control, but also on ways to minimize its impact while ongoing transmission occurs.

With the experience of the SARS epidemic in 2003, we have further fine-tuned the various public health measures. Hong Kong's preparedness planning adopts a cross-sectoral and multidisciplinary approach. A number of drills and exercises related to infectious diseases including avian influenza have been conducted since 2004 to test the workability of the plan and to familiarize the government departments and other agencies of their respective roles. The gaps so identified are valuable feedback for refining the plans.

In February 2005, a Preparedness Plan for Influenza Pandemic was developed based on WHO's guidelines and recommendations. It outlines the government's emergency preparedness on a three-tiered coordination response system — Alert, Serious and Emergency Levels — based on different risk-graded epidemiological scenarios relevant to Hong Kong. All government departments as well as private sector organizations have been requested to develop their own contingency plans with reference to the three-tier response levels to ensure consistent enhancement of measures in respective settings.

Each response level prescribes a clear command and control structure and a given set of public health actions required (details are available on the CHP website).[f] A brief overview is summarized in the ensuing paragraphs.

---

[f]CHP website at www.chp.gov.hk

Alert Response Level
*Alert Response Level (ARL) will be activated when either there is/are confirmed human case(s) of avian influenza **outside** Hong Kong; or upon confirmation of highly pathogenic avian influenza (HPAI) outbreaks in poultry populations **outside** Hong Kong; or confirmation of HPAI **in** Hong Kong in imported birds in quarantine, in wild birds, in recreational parks, in pet bird shops or in the natural environment.*

A significant public health objective is to prevent introduction of the disease into Hong Kong and to detect local cases as early as practicable. Undoubtedly, port health measures form the first line of defence in protecting Hong Kong. At ARL, temperature checking by infra-red devices is arranged for inbound travellers at all immigration control points, including land borders, sea ports and the airport, to detect individuals with symptoms and reduce the spread of the disease early. Though the effectiveness of border temperature checks may be limited because avian influenza patients can be infectious even before developing fever, medicals posts are set up at the airport, ports and border points to watch for travelers displaying symptoms of infectious diseases.

A targeted intervention approach is used whereby on-flight health announcements are instituted on flights originating from affected areas. For outbound travelers to affected areas, health advice is given by distributing health materials at airline counters. Scenario plans and protocols for suspected avian influenza cases arriving on flights are developed and tested.

An effective and sensitive surveillance system is important in order to capture any human case which may somehow evade detection and enter into Hong Kong. In this regard, Hong Kong has listed Influenza A (H5, H7 and H9) as statutorily notifiable infectious diseases since 2004 and healthcare professionals can conveniently submit notifications through a web-based platform newly setup in March 2005.

The disease surveillance system must also be comprehensive to reflect the overall local situation. Apart from the influenza-like illness reporting sentinels established in over 100 public and private clinics, fever and absenteeism reporting have also commenced in elderly homes and childcare centers through a voluntary scheme. Swift investigations and interventions are enabled through monitoring for any unusual trends of influenza-like illness in the community. Hospital surveillance on pneumonia and staff sickness reporting, and laboratory surveillance on influenza virus typing provides further support.

> **Serious Response Level**
> *Serious Response Level will be activated upon confirmation of human case(s) of avian influenza **in** Hong Kong **without** evidence of efficient human-to-human transmission; or confirmation of HPAI outbreaks in the environment of or among poultry population in retail markets, wholesale markets or farms **in** Hong Kong due to a strain with known human health impact. A Steering Committee chaired by the Secretary for Health, Welfare and Food will be set up to steer government responses.*

When human cases are detected locally, either imported or infected from poultry, Hong Kong has a narrow window of opportunity to contain the disease as soon as possible, identify foci of infection and prevent local transmission and exportation of the disease to other places. Aggressive public health interventions have to be adopted, including stringent health screening measures of temperature checks and health declarations at all entry and exit points. All close contacts of avian influenza patients would be barred from leaving Hong Kong during the home confinement period.

In deciding on the most appropriate disease prevention measures to be taken, the Government will have full regard on the prevailing situation of the outbreak(s) in Hong Kong and neighboring regions, mode of epidemic transmission and efficiency, scale of spreading and incubation period, the latest scientific evidence, etc. as well as WHO's recommendations and the International Health Regulations (IHR). There should be a proper balance between effective disease prevention and smooth flow of passengers and goods. If necessary, for instance, travellers will be advised to postpone non-essential travel to affected areas in accordance with WHO travel advices, if any.

With the lack of effective pandemic influenza vaccines, antivirals such as neuramindase inhibitors become one of the weapons for treatment of infected patients or prophylaxis for contacts, healthcare workers and other essential service providers, and workers involved in culling operations. Hong Kong is stockpiling antiviral drugs at a target level of over 20 million doses. This is based on the local pandemic influenza experience in 1968, during which around 15% of the population were infected.

Aggressive outbreak response measures will be put in place with a view to achieving total control of the disease before the virus acquires efficient human-to-human transmission capability. Epidemiological investigations and contact tracing will be conducted. Close contacts will be put into confinement, and social contacts will be put under medical surveillance for a period consistent with the incubation period of the disease. If there are two or more suspected or confirmed cases detected, a multidisciplinary response team will be set up to carry out investigations and advice on disinfection of the affected premises.

Dispersion of cases over the territory will pose difficulty in epidemic control. Moreover, infectious cases may come into contact with other types of patients in certain settings such as at Accident and Emergency Departments of hospitals, which potentially pose infectious risk to other patients. To minimize such risk, some clinics will be turned into designated centers for fever cases, and suspected avian influenza patients can then receive initial management at a nearby designated clinic.

Emergency Response Level

*The Emergency Response Level (ERL) will be activated when there is evidence confirming efficient human-to-human transmission of novel influenza occurring **overseas** or in Hong Kong; or when WHO formally declares that the world is entering pandemic phase. It represents a turning point in epidemic control. The Chief Executive will chair the inter-departmental Steering Committee as the overall commander.*

As the number of cases accumulates, the government will review the hospital capacity and determine if the hospitals should only provide essential medical service and transfer non-urgent medical services such as minor operations to private hospitals or clinics.

Social distancing interventions at the community level, such as closure of schools or certain public places, will be enforced if epidemiological, clinical and virological investigations reveal that such settings facilitate ongoing spread of the disease. For example, school closure is thus a way to minimize transmission amongst school children.

The challenge of advising and implementing community interventions lies in the paucity of concrete scientific evidence on their effectiveness, practicability and their acceptance by the public, as well as political and social impact. Moreover, social distancing interventions, when prolonged, could have profound and prolonged social and economic impact.

It is also imperative to slow down progression of the epidemic and minimize loss of human lives in order to buy time for the production of an effective vaccine. Development of vaccine for a novel influenza virus may take as long as six months. Combination of antivirals for treatment or prophylaxis, and infection control measures, including isolation and quarantine, will continue to be used for outbreak control in the initial period of the

ERL. The government will closely monitor the supply of antivirals while at the same time proactively keeping track of the development of global vaccines to ensure rapid access.

There is a possibility that at a late phase of ERL, a huge number of cases may simply render the isolation and confinement arrangements unable to be further sustained. Nonetheless, with the support and cooperation of the mass community in good compliance on wearing surgical masks, hand-washing and healthy lifestyle, each individual can be an effective mobile "quarantine unit" even in the absence of confinement.

Epilogue

Preparedness for avian influenza is a challenging issue. Given ongoing virus evolution, we do not know when and where a mutation or reassortment event that happens will confer the H5N1 virus the ability to pass efficiently from human to human. Human history indicates that influenza pandemic will occur on a periodic basis, and 37 years have passed since the last pandemic in 1968. With globalization, it is unrealistic to predict that Hong Kong can be free from the disease should a pandemic occur. Yet certainly, it is only those who prepared well can respond well; and only those who respond well can minimize the impact of the outbreak, for the good of the public and the world. Let us continue to join hands to guard against the threat of avian influenza, or for that matter the influenza pandemic. Effective health protection always starts with individuals; a healthy lifestyle, good personal hygiene and handwashing are the fundamentals.

15

Singapore's Efforts and Experiences in Influenza Control

Paul A. Tambyah

Singapore is a global city in Southeast Asia and thus has been a major point of intersection for influenza transmission throughout history. As many other authors in this volume have pointed out, it is thought that many influenza pandemics have arisen out of the backyard farms of Southeast Asia and have been amplified in the crowded cities of East Asia before spreading rapidly worldwide. While there is no evidence that this occurred in 1918 with the most lethal influenza pandemic of all, this probably occurred with the "Asian Flu" of 1957 and the "Hongkong Flu" of 1968. With current outbreaks of H5N1 in birds in many parts of East Asia as well as sporadic cases of H5N1 influenza in humans, there is the concern that once again Singapore or any of the other major cities of Southeast or East Asia will become the starting point for the worldwide dissemination of pandemic influenza.

Surveillance

The first step in control of any emerging infectious disease is to know that it exists and to answer the basic questions that every epidemiologist asks: What? Where? When? And How? These are the goals of surveillance systems that have been established over the years. The World Health Organization

(WHO) established a system of surveillance sites for the early detection of novel strains of influenza soon after the Second World War. These are credited with clarifying the spread of the 1957 and 1968 pandemic influenza strains. They are also responsible for the detection of circulating strains of seasonal influenza which are reported to WHO which then decides which strains will go into the influenza vaccine for the coming year. The influenza virus has on its surface, a number of markers, predominantly the well-known H (or hemagglutinin) and N (or neuraminidase) which currently are only H3N2 or H1N1. However, due to a process of antigenic drift, every year, the H3N2 and H1N1 might vary slightly and thus the vaccine from the previous year might not protect an individual from the flu strain that is circulating in the current year. Thus, the WHO influenza surveillance sites provide vital information for planning for influenza vaccination even for regular seasonal influenza. Singapore has been part of this global influenza surveillance system since the 1970s and in 1972, Singapore General Hospital's Department of Pathology was designated the National Influenza Center by WHO.

The 1957 Asian Flu Pandemic

Perhaps the best illustration of Singapore's experiences in control of influenza is Singapore's response to the 1957 Asian flu pandemic. In retrospect, this pandemic is now thought to have started in China and thence through Hongkong, Singapore and Russia to the rest of the world. Researchers at the University of Malaya in Singapore led by Professor Lim Kok Ann published one of the earliest descriptions of the epidemiology and virology of the the pandemic in the *Lancet* in 1957.[1] In fact, the reference strain H2N2/A/Singapore/1/57 isolated at the university laboratories in Singapore have remained the reference strains for researchers all over the world till today. Professor Lim and his team studied workers at the Naval Base in Singapore. They were able to document an outbreak in 298 patients (including both workers and their dependents) who were admitted to hospital. Thirty-nine had complications, predominantly pneumonia and these occurred mainly in the older patients as well as young children. Striking findings included the observation that influenza tended to occur more in younger individuals and that Asians had a higher attack rate than Europeans — probably because they were younger. Professor Lim and his colleagues also noted that the peak incidence of disease in workers was a few days before the peak in dependents suggesting that workers were infected at work and they brought the infection home. In addition to the hospitalized patients at the Naval Base hospital, Prof. Lim and colleagues noted that in the second week of May, the number of new cases at the outpatient clinic at the General Hospital reached as high as 1000 new cases a day compared with a baseline figure of less than 100. There were three peaks, the first from 7–9 May with 800–1000 new outpatient cases a day, the second from 12–17 May with 300–700 new cases a day and a final smaller spurt on 20 May before the epidemic tapered off. Because the epidemic seemed to taper off on its own, there were no drastic measures that needed to be taken or could be taken in time to control the outbreak. In addition, as Prof. Lim notes in his report, although the mortality rate was increased by the pandemic, the majority of deaths occurred in older individuals with chronic diseases. Drs. Yeoh and Dourado of the pediatric unit at the Singapore General Hospital also documented the impact of the 1957 pandemic of influenza and they recorded an increase in both admissions (a doubling of inpatient admissions during the second week of May) as well as deaths among children with more than 40 deaths per week during the two weeks of the outbreak compared with a baseline of ten to 20 deaths a week. In their report in the *British Medical Journal* of 1957,[2] Drs. Yeoh and Dourado documented that 1231 children were admitted to the hospital pediatric unit during the epidemic period of whom 196 died. Post-mortem examinations were obtained for 175 of them and the majority of the deaths were due to pneumonia with occasional involvement of the gastrointestinal tract.

Dr. B. R. Sreenivasan, writing in the *Proceedings of the Alumni Association of Malaya* wrote,[3] "This epidemic found us unprepared. The medical profession should have a machinery whereby early on in an epidemic, representatives of the profession can get together in order to decide: (1) how best the sick can be dealt with, (2) what propaganda should be done to prevent the spread of the disease, and (3) how best the epidemic can be studied from the epidemiologic, bacteriological and clinical points of view. Such a machinery can be brought into existence if there is one professional body representative of all medical interests throughout the country." He subsequently went on to become the founder president of the Singapore Medical Association. It is interesting that just as SARS spun off improved infection control and hospital epidemiology in Singapore hospitals, the 1957 Asian flu pandemic led at least in part to the formation of a professional body of doctors determined to take action to deal with future pandemic threats among other issues.

In summary, the major response to the 1957 Asian flu pandemic in Singapore was scientific. Careful surveillance in the segment of the population that was accessible to Western medical care was the cornerstone of case detection. This was difficult for then as now; many Singaporeans depend on traditional medicine especially for coughs, colds and upper respiratory tract infections. Professor Lim commented that the lower attack rates in Asian women in his study could be due to the fact that at that time, many Asian women did not consult "Western-trained" physicians. Although the role of "Western" medicine has increased considerably in Singapore, it is clear that if surveillance for influenza-like illness in Singapore and most Asian countries is to be comprehensive, we have to engage practitioners of traditional and alternative medicine. This will be a challenge as there is a considerable lack of understanding on both sides that will have to be overcome. The work of University and Government Clinician Scientists in documenting the Asian Flu outbreak in 1957 in leading medical journals exemplifies Singapore's integrated approach to medical research involving academics, scientists, clinicians across institutions and public health professionals. In recent years, Singapore has once again seen tremendous investment in biomedical science and research and it is hoped that once again, Singapore scientists and clinicians will be at the forefront of research into the next pandemic influenza should it occur.

The 1968 Hong Kong Flu Pandemic

In 1968, the most recent pandemic of influenza, again, Singapore responded strongly with good science and creative surveillance. In back-to-back papers published in the *Singapore Medical Journal*, Dr. Kadri of the University of Singapore's Health Service[4] and Dr. Mary Yin-Murphy[5] described both the epidemiology and the virology of the 1968 Hong Kong flu pandemic in Singapore. Dr. Kadri reported on 965 cases of influenza presenting to the University Health Service at the University of Singapore during four weeks in August–September 1968. What is striking about his report is that the attack rate of this novel strain of influenza was around 15% for university students but as high as 36% among the non-academic staff of the the university. He made the comment that the non-academic staff tended to come from the lower socio-economic groups and suggested that that might be the reason for the higher attack rate in that group. Dr. Yin-Murphy's paper describes virological and serological results which demonstrated that the cause of the pandemic was indeed a novel strain of influenza due to an antigenic shift. None of the tested individuals had any baseline immunity to the new strain. The results also showed that it was the same strain that had first emerged in Hongkong in the month prior.

Professor Wong Hock Boon reported on the epidemic in children in an article in the *Journal of the Singapore Pediatric Society*.[6] Once again in 1968, as with the 1957 Asian flu pandemic, there was a rise in the number of admissions to the pediatric department with a rise at the peak of the out-break to 300–350 cases from around 150–200 cases a week. Professor Wong reviewed 140 cases of which 47 had proven influenza either by culture or serology or both. Again, the majority of these were from one to five years of age. Ten of the 140 children died; the majority very quickly, within two days of admission. This is important as it suggests that the children died of the influenza pneumonia or pneumonitis (another kind of lung inflammation) due to the virus itself and not due to secondary bacterial infection. Some have speculated that the high mortality in the 1918 pandemic was due to the fact that there were no antibiotics in use at the time. In 1968, penicillin and some of the other early generation antibiotics were in widespread use but influenza still claimed the lives of vulnerable young children.

The major contributions of Singapore's response to the 1968 pandemic influenza were thus the recognition once again that relatively contained institutions such as the university were a good focal point for understanding the epidemiology of the disease as well as the importance of understanding the way the disease affects children.

Education

In addition to responding to influenza pandemics, Singapore's medical and scientific leadership have always felt the responsibility to educate the community at large and the local medical fraternity in particular about the latest scientific and clinical developments in influenza. These efforts date all the way back to 1937, soon after the causative agent of influenza was determined to be a "filterable agent" or virus by the work of Dr. Shope. Dr. P. N. Bardhan, a local graduate of Singapore's own King Edward VII College of Medicine wrote in the *Malayan Medical Journal*[7] about the clinical and laboratory features of influenza. He commented that "all upper respiratory infections are not influenza; in fact most are not." This is an idea which many infectious disease physicians try to this day to communicate to patients and caregivers alike. A "cold" is **not** the "flu." The "flu" kills people, especially the elderly and very young children. A cold might give you the sniffles but without the fever, muscle aches, lethargy that characterizes influenza, you are unlikely to run into serious complications.

Inter-pandemic Surveillance and Modeling

We have not had an influenza pandemic since 1968. Since then, Singapore has continued to be a WHO surveillance center and we are part of the WHO influenza network which is responsible for contributing virus isolates from the selected polyclinics. These make up part of the decision making process into what goes into the seasonal influenza vaccine every year around the world. Singapore's Ministry of Health also monitors acute respiratory infections at polyclinics and influenza and pneumonia deaths. These data were recently analyzed and published in the *Emerging Infectious Diseases* journal.[8] Dr. Angela Chow and her colleagues at the Ministry of Health report that, annually, approximately 580 excess deaths in Singapore are attributable to influenza. Overall, the death rate from influenza is comparable to that in subtropical and temperate countries. The authors commented that despite the Ministry of Health encouraging influenza vaccination for those aged over 65 since 2003, the uptake of vaccination is low with less than 10% coverage of this group. They make a strong case for strengthening Singapore's public health efforts to control the effects of seasonal or "regular" influenza pointing out that SARS caused 33 deaths but galvanized the nation while influenza causes more than 500 deaths a year but is still largely "under the radar screen."

Pandemic Preparedness

In addition to responding to "regular" or "seasonal" influenza, Singapore's public health community is actively engaged in preparing for the possibility of pandemic influenza. Singapore's Ministry of Health has published a pandemic influenza plan which is available online at the Ministry's website (http://www.moh.gov.sg/cmaweb/attachments/topic/36c564c023S0/MainDec05.pdf). This is a very comprehensive plan which details Singapore's response to an influenza pandemic. This is a multi-agency plan which involves an impressive array of governmental agencies from the Cabinet through the Ministries of Information and Communications, Home Affairs, Environment and Water, National Development, Education and a host of others. The lead agency will be the Ministry of Health and surveillance is the keystone of the initial response. This is a mix of virological and community-based surveillance using the system established since 1973. The plan also addresses the prioritizing of vaccination when it becomes available as well as the stockpile of oseltamivir which is believed to have some benefit in reducing the severity of influenza or possibly preventing infections in some settings. Some controversial aspects of the plan include the idea of designating one hospital as the main influenza treatment hospital — a strategy not employed in the successful management of the 1957 and 1968 pandemics. This is presumably based on the use of this strategy during the SARS epidemic. Lessons learned from that epidemic on the need to severely restrict the inter-hospital transfer of patients to limit the inter-hospital spread of infection will hopefully be taken into consideration. Other controversial aspects of the plan include the possible use of quarantine and border controls, again based on the possible success of this strategy during SARS. WHO's working group has published a review of non-pharmaceutical strategies for the control of pandemic influenza in which they reviewed the experience of quarantine and border controls during previous epidemics of influenza. In Africa and Australia, because of the relative geographic isolation of many communities, attempts were made to quarantine and isolate communities during the 1918 pandemic. Similar efforts took place in Israel and South Africa in 1957 but more for political reasons. These were not successful in keeping pandemic influenza from these areas and the conclusion of the authors is that quarantine and border controls are likely to be futile once a pandemic is established. In the unlikely eventuality that Singapore is the starting point for a new global pandemic of influenza, there is the possibility that quarantine might be a useful strategy for the containment of this novel strain.

The Singapore approach to pandemic influenza preparedness has three desired outcomes (1) maintenance of essential services and minimizing the disruption of normal life on the island, (2) reducing mortality and morbidity by treatment of all cases with influenza-like illness, and (3) slowing and limiting the spread of influenza by a combination of border health, hospital infection control and community measures such as possible closing of schools and limiting public events.

These strategies are based on WHO's guidelines for pandemic influenza planning. WHO has come up with a checklist for pandemic influenza planning which they suggest that their member states should consider in preparing for a pandemic. The checklist is also very comprehensive and includes (1) command and control infrastructure, (2) modeling of the various scenarios, (3) developing a communications plan and engaging the media, (4) establishing a mechanism for communication with healthcare facilities, (5) assessing the legal framework for measures that need to be taken during a pandemic, (6) establishing a comprehensive surveillance system to detect upper respiratory tract infections, influenza virus circulating as well as clusters of unusual illnesses, (7) strengthening laboratory diagnostic facilities and establishing laboratory protocols, (8) developing protocols for epidemiologic investigations, (9) clinical management protocols, and (10) use of antivirals, vaccines, community measures and perhaps most importantly to an academic infectious disease physician, developing a research agenda to study the consequences of the various actions taken during the pandemic. All these are also available online at the WHO website at http://www.who.int/csr/resources/publications/influenza/WHO_CDS_CSR_GIP_2005_4/en/.

Both Singapore's and WHO's plans focus on different alert levels. These are based somewhat loosely on the concept popularized by the US "Homeland Security" system. An alert level of green or yellow is generally thought to indicate a low risk of a pandemic and the measures that are recommended are thus appropriately restrained. At the levels red or black, there is thought to be widespread death and economic devastation along the lines described in D. A. Fisher's chapter in this volume. At that point, there is no rationale for doing any kind of border health or screening surveillance as almost everyone everywhere would have been exposed to the virus and is either recovering and immune or dead and dying. There are of course intermediate levels in both schemes. It is interesting to note that they differ on the definitions of these levels. At the time of writing, Singapore is at alert level Green 1 which is defined as "isolated local or external cases of animal to human case, but the threat of human-to-human infection remains low." In contrast, WHO currently (30 January 2006) is at alert level Yellow 3 which indicates no or very limited human-to-human transmission. The distinction is important as Singapore's plan calls for major activities to commence at alert level Yellow including limitation of inter-hospital transfer and intensified healthcare worker surveillance. I personally think that Singapore's approach is more pragmatic as there is a very real danger of over-reacting to the threat of pandemic influenza.

Over-reacting?

The best illustration of an "over-reaction" to the threat of pandemic influenza is what has been described as the "Swine Flu Episode" in the United States in 1976. In the summer of that year, a number of soldiers in New Jersey came down with a novel strain of influenza. At least one of them died. There was a great deal of anxiety about a pandemic emerging the coming winter. A vaccine was rushed into production and in an unprecedented public health effort, 45 million Americans were vaccinated. Unfortunately, a small number of them suffered a rare complication of that particular influenza vaccine — the Guillain Barre Syndrome. There were also no further cases of the novel strain of influenza beyond that small cluster at the Army Camp in New Jersey. In other words, a pandemic did not occur and a number of people suffered from a side effect of vaccination. There is still a considerable debate about the decisions that were made during that public health campaign and the role of the media and those who were more concerned about the political implications rather than the science of the disease. There are a number of articles in the January issue of the *Emerging Infectious Diseases* journal which are available online at http://www.cdc.gov/ncidod/EID/vol12no01/contents_v12n01.htm. These are worth reading for anyone who is involved in the decision making process for pandemic influenza planning. It is hoped that Singapore and the world's response to pandemic influenza is guided primarily by science. One of my Indonesian colleagues, Dr. Sardikin Giriputro who is the deputy director of the Sulianti Saroso Infectious Disease Hospital in Jakarta put it very well. He said, "If there is a pandemic, hopefully, we will be prepared. If there is no pandemic, local capabilities and resources will be upgraded a notch." Either way, communities, hospitals and institutions can only benefit from a thorough, scientific evidence-based approach to pandemic influenza planning.

Acknowledgments

I would like to thank Mrs. Mercedes Cheong of the Medical Library, NUS, for her resourcefulness in obtaining some of the historical references.

References

1. Lim KA, Smith A, Hale JH, Glass J. Influenza outbreak in Singapore. *Lancet* 1957;ii:791–796.
2. Yeoh OS, Dourado H. Influenza epidemic in Singapore children. Clinical impressions. *Br Med J* 1957;29:1253–1255.
3. Sreenivasan BR. The recent influenza epidemic in Singapore. *Proc Alum Assn Malaya* 1957;10:211–215.
4. Kadri ZN. An outbreak of "Hong Kong Flu" in Singapore. Part 1: Clinical study. *Sing Med J* 1970;11:30–32.
5. Yin-Murphy M. An outbreak of "Hong Kong Flu" in Singapore. Part 2: Virological and serological report. *Sing Med J* 1970;11:33–37.
6. Wong HB. A clinical study of proved cases of influenza affecting children. *J Sing Pediatr Soc* 1969;11:108–114.
7. Bardhan PN. Notes on etiology and diagnosis of influenza. *Malayan Med J* 1937;1:114–115.
8. Chow A, Ma S, Ling AE, Chew SK. Influenza associated deaths in tropical Singapore. *Emerg Infect Dis* 2006;12(1):114–121.

16

Influenza, the Rockefeller Institute and, "The Swine Flu Episode^a, 1976"

Richard M. Krause

Introduction/Summary

The editors have asked that I describe my observations concerning the threat of a possible swine flu epidemic in 1976, and, as Director of the National Institute of Allergy and Infectious Diseases (NIAID), my role in the public health surveillance (PHS) response to this threat.

The swine flu outbreak at Fort Dix, New Jersey in the winter of 1976 was due to H1N1, and the concern at the time was that this virus was most likely a direct descendent of the influenza strain that caused the pandemic of 1918. This conclusion was based on the presence of antibodies to the H1N1 antigens in the survivors of the 1918 flu pandemic and the belief that the 1918 virus eventually was transmitted to pigs of the Midwest where it has persisted, and where it has caused sporadic human cases. Had it broken out of the pig stye, so to speak, and caused the outbreak in humans at Fort Dix?

In view of these events in February of '76, the decision was made by PHS to prepare an influenza vaccine with the Fort Dix strain and immunize a large segment of the US population. This was achieved by October of that

---

^aEpisode: From the Greek, *Epeisodion*, a part in an ancient tragedy between two choric songs.

year. I agreed with that decision. Why? This essay is my effort to answer that question.

I came to the NIH in November 1975 after 20 years at Rockefeller University where my research was in microbiology and immunology, but not virology. But from my years at Rockefeller, I had a rich exposure to the lore of influenza research in that institution that extended back to World War I and the 1918 influenza pandemic. Central to my reflections is the research of Dr. Thomas Francis and others at the Rockefeller University over many decades. Recorded here also is my store of general knowledge about influenza at the time I became Director of NIAID.

We are now faced with the threat of a possible influenza pandemic due to bird flu H5N1. Many who must now make wise decisions about the public health response will not be virologists or flu experts, as I was not, and they will need to base their decisions on the opinion of the experts *and* on their own scientific evaluation of the facts of the case.

I hope my reflections here on what I knew in 1976 about influenza — what I brought to the table as is said today — will be useful for those who must decide the PHS response to the threat of H5N1 in 2005. They have my best wishes and good luck.

————oo————

Thomas Francis began his 1953 lecture "Influenza: The *Newe Acquayantance*" with these reflections on the history of the disease.

> "Maye it please your Honor immediately upon the Queen's arrival here, she fell acquainted with a new disease that is common in this town, called here the *Newe Acquayantance*, which passed also throughe her whole Courte, neither sparing lordes, ladies nor damoysells, not so much as either Frenche or English ... There was no appearance of danger, nor manie that die of the disease, excepte some olde folks. I am ashamed to say that I have byne free of it, seeing it seketh acquayantance at all man's handes."

> Written in a letter in 1562 by Sir Thomas Randolph,
> Ambassador from Queen Elizabeth I to the Court of
> Mary, Queen of Scots, Edinburgh, to Cecil in London.[1]

"The statement serves to recall the fact that, over and over in its long career, an extensive prevalence of influenza has been hailed as a new disease ... and in various popular names — the jolly rant, the new delight, gallants' disease, the fashionable illness, and, as now, the flu or, more fashionably, this virus thing," in French *La Grippe*.

"On the other hand, the fact that the occurrences attracted considerable attention of many of the outstanding physicians during centuries in which severe disease and high mortality were commonplace indicates that there were qualities which distinguished them from other contemporary disturbances. Certain of them are repeated almost constantly in the chronicles. The sudden appearance, with the rapid, widespread involvement of all ages and kinds, is one of them. Sir Thomas Willis, outstanding epidemiologist and clinician, describes the onset in 1658:

> "About the end of April, suddenly a Distemper arose, as if sent by some blast of the stars, which laid hold on very many together: that in some towns, in the space of a week, above a thousand people fell sick together.
>   Then the feature of low mortality is prominent. The epidemic of 1580 has been called the first real pandemic, involving Asia, Europe and Africa extensively. T. Short states: 'This disease raged all over Europe at least, and prevailed for six weeks ... Though all had it, few died in these countries, except such as were let blood of, or had unsound viscera'."[1]

I recall reading in 1953 this paper The *Newe Acquayantance* by Thomas Francis, Jr.[1] when I was a house officer on W. Barry Wood's service at Barnes Hospital, St. Louis. One of our responsibilities was to read the current literature and select reading assignments for the medical student clerks on the ward, so that they were well primed for the professor's bedside rounds. I assigned this paper to the students. I have not read it again until I was preparing this commentary. On reflection I wish I had done so at the time of the swine flu episode in 1976. I believe I would have had greater insight into the possible threat of a flu pandemic. Certainly Francis' lecture and his conclusions and speculations about the mysteries of 1918 influenza should temper our strategies for coping with a possible human pandemic arising like some phoenix from the current flu epidemic in Asian chickens.

In 1918, my parents and my brothers, then children, were living in a small town in southeastern Ohio. When I was a teenager in the 1930s, I recall my mother's reflections on the influenza pandemic. There was in addition the mobilization for war. It was general knowledge in 1918 that influenza was an infectious disease, but as yet of unknown cause. Recall the 20th century began with the well established and accepted fact that many contagious diseases were due to specific microbes, but at the time there was no specific treatment for any of them except syphilis and malaria. So there was widespread anxiety and alarm.

Our home was near a chair factory, and after work many of the employees walked past our house. From time to time they would spit either phlegm or tobacco juice on the pavement. For such occasions, my Mother always had a tea kettle of boiling water so she could immediately scald the "damned spot" in the hope that this would kill the unknown and unseen germs that were causing influenza, the better to protect my two young brothers from catching "the bug." I relate this personal anecdote just to remind you that even in the 1930s when I was a teenager, the 1918 pandemic was still a living memory. To this day, that pandemic casts the longest shadow, although it is likely the AIDS pandemic will take its place.

My next experience with influenza was in 1944 when I was in the US Army. The flu vaccine had just been developed by Francis, Salk and others. Their work had been supported by the US Army under the auspices of the Armed Forces Epidemiology Board (AFEB). 1918 was still fresh in their memory. Fifty thousand soldiers had died of influenza. We GIs were lined up at the dispensary and given the vaccine, one soldier right after the other, with the same 50 ml syringe, although as I recall the needles were changed, or at least wiped clean (if not sterilized) with 70% alcohol. The discovery of serum hepatitis had been made in Germany about the same time, but this information had not yet filtered through to the medical community in the US. I have wondered since then how much hepatitis occurred as a result of that first mass flu immunization of the US Army.

I recall to this day the moderately severe local reaction, swelling, considerable tenderness, and pain at the site of the flu inoculation. Also many had systemic reactions. I remember that the vaccine in the syringe was turbid.

I did not know then that the vaccine had been grown in eggs. I have wondered since then if the turbidity of the vaccine was due to a residue of chicken feathers! Clearly purification had a long way to go in 1944. I have been taking the influenza vaccine yearly for several decades, and with the new purified vaccines I have been free of local reactions.

There was no more exciting place to pursue medical research than the O. T. Avery Laboratory when Thomas Francis arrived at the Rockefeller Institute for Medical Research in 1928 where he worked until 1938, first on pneumococcal pneumonia, and then on influenza. By 1918 Avery had been successful in developing anti-pneumococcal serum therapy, and reported highly successful results. In his hands mortality dropped from 30%–35% to 4% with specific anti-pneumococcal serum. No surprise that the Rockefeller Hospital staff had been mobilized to help in World War I to combat influenza and pneumonia.

There is another important aspect about the history of the Rockefeller Institute and the 1918 influenza epidemic that should be recounted here. This concerns the identification of hemolytic streptococci as one of the causes of secondary bronchopneumonia in influenza patients during the pandemic.[b] At the time the bacterial etiology of this complication in influenza patients was clouded in uncertainty.

Antiserum was still the treatment of choice for pneumococcal pneumonia when Francis came in 1928. Furthermore, the chemical specificity of the capsular polysaccharides had been established. Still to come was the discovery of C-reactive protein and an alternative to serum therapy. Francis was to work on both of these projects, and then later on influenza.

---

[b]When the Rockefeller Hospital physicians were mobilized for the World War I effort, several were sent to Fort Sam Houston, Texas, including Alphonse Dochez, now a captain in the Army, and O. T. Avery, then a Private in the US Army because at the time he was a Canadian citizen. Later a citizen, he was promoted to officer rank. Rebecca Craighill (later Lancefield) was a technical assistant at the time.

They went to Fort Sam Houston to investigate pneumonia in military recruits. That they did, but what emerged was also of great importance and entirely unexpected. A 1919 paper documented the discovery that hemolytic streptococci, later identified by Rebecca Lancefield as Group A, were the cause of many cases of secondary pneumonia in the influenza patients. In the initial 1918 study, hemolytic streptococci were divisible into four types.[2] An unknown antigen in each type stimulated type-specific immunity in mice. At the time, there was no clear picture as to the nature of the antigens which induced such immunity. What was clear was that they were completely unlike "specific soluble substance" of the pneumococci. Ten years later, working with the Ft. Sam Houston strains, Lancefield showed that type-specific immunity in humans was due to the immune response to type-specific M proteins.[3] She also showed that all the M types belonged to Group A which have a distinctive carbohydrate antigen, and the cause of most streptococcal infections including pharyngitis, impetigo, and scarlet fever. Of great importance was the subsequent discovery that *only* Group A streptococcal pharyngitis caused rheumatic fever.

In an article written immediately after Francis's death, Colin M. MacLeod recalled:[4]

"On coming to Avery's laboratory, Francis and William Tillett worked together on cutaneous and serological reactions to products of pneumococcus, particularly the specific capsular polysaccharides and the 'C' or somatic carbohydrate, now known to be a constituent of the bacterial cell wall. Over the three-year period of their collaboration two remarkable findings came forth.

The first of these was that there occurs in the blood of patients with many acute infections a new substance, not an antibody in the usual sense, which reacts specifically with the 'C' carbohydrate of pneumococcus to give a precipitation reaction. During recovery from the disease the 'C-reactive protein,' as it came to be known, diminishes in amount and within a few days disappears entirely. This is an enigmatic reaction whose function in man and animals is still unknown, but which provides a useful clinical test to measure the activity of a variety of infectious processes, for example the activity of the inflammatory process in rheumatic fever.

Francis and Tillett also discovered that minute amounts of specific capsular polysaccharides of pneumococcus injected intracutaneously in man cause the development of specific antibodies and that the antibodies are protective ..., an observation pursued by Robert Austrian that would lead to a successful pneumococcal vaccine.

While Francis was in Avery's laboratory, René Dubos and Avery had developed their famous studies on an induced enzyme obtained from a soil bacterium which specifically hydrolyzes the capsular polysaccharide of pneumococcus Type III whether the latter is in solution or attached to the living, virulent pneumococcus."

MacLeod went on to say:

"Francis, with Terrell, devised methods for producing Type III pneumonia in monkeys and published meticulous studies of its clinical course. In collaboration with Dubos and Avery they then went on to demonstrate in this experimental disease of primates, which simulates pneumococcal pneumonia in man, that the SIII enzyme has striking curative properties.

Unfortunately, a test of the therapeutic effect in man was never carried out, because the sulfa drugs were introduced shortly thereafter, a highly successful treatment of many infections including pneumococcal pneumonia; the first of the wonder drugs."

A young scientist could hardly have been more productive than was Francis in his early years at Rockefeller, so it is not entirely clear why he phased out his pneumococcal research and sought out other opportunities in virology. Perhaps he was baffled, even frustrated by the vagaries of his early work on the pneumococcal transformation experiments. There is no publication describing his efforts on transformation. Perhaps he was seeking an independent line of research. True or not, John Paul relates Francis' recollection about his early years in Avery's lab, and his emerging interests in virology.[5]

"Somewhere in these early days, I rode on the train from New York to Princeton, New Jersey, with two leaders in virology: Thomas Rivers and Christopher Andrews to see a third, Dick Shope. In those days, virology had not yet descended to the level of the common man, and I listened as a privileged young man to their sage and effete comments on viruses and their behavior."

Whatever the reason, Francis withdrew from the pneumonia service at Rockefeller, and began his work there on influenza. In 1934 he published in *Science* a report on the transmission of influenza by a filterable virus.[6]

This brings me then to Francis' research on influenza and the development of the flu vaccine. His work has been well summarized by Sir Charles Stuart-Harris. In earlier years he and Francis had worked together on various matters pertaining to influenza. I quote Sir Charles, written some 35 years after he had collaborated with Dr. Francis in New York:[7]

"Of all the achievements for which Dr. Thomas Francis will be remembered, none surpasses his contributions to the elucidation of the problem of influenza. As the first American to recover and to study influenza virus in the laboratory, Dr. Francis lit in his own hand the torch of discovery which still burns brightly in the hands of others. *When the first evidence of antigenic variation of the influenza A viruses was published in 1936 by Dr. Thomas Magill and Dr. Francis, it was received with incredulity by the London team of influenza workers of the Medical Research Council, Dr. Christopher Andrewes, Wilson Smith and Patrick Laidlaw. The latter, however, examined their viruses by neu-*tralization with a *hyperimmune horse serum* whereas the Rockefeller workers used a more *specific rabbit serum. On such apparently small* *differences may turn matters of great moment, and the great importance both epidemiologically and immunologically of the antigenic diversity of both influenza viruses A and B is now recognized universally.*

Dr. Francis's demonstration that subcutaneous immunization with influenza vaccine can protect against epidemic influenza was an equally significant finding."

In 1944 Francis *et al.*[8] demonstrated the protective effect of vaccination against influenza A in volunteers. This led to the Army's successful influenza vaccination program that same year. His discovery of antigenic variation of influenza A virus had fundamental implications for the development of an influenza vaccine.

In the 1950s and '60s, at the annual AFEB meeting, the Army and the Navy presented each year the results on influenza prevention with the vaccine then in use. There was, of course, the yearly modification of the vaccine because of the emergence of shift and drift in influenza virus antigenic composition. The military data were always in support of the efficacy of the influenza vaccine, recognizing, of course, this was being given to healthy, young recruits and servicemen between the ages of 18 and 45. In those earlier years, the vaccine formulation for the military had a higher content of inactivated virus than did the preparation for civilian use. If I recall there were a somewhat greater number of local reactions at the site of injection with the military vaccine than with the civilian one. But as was noted, the military preparation was very effective in preventing influenza in the troops, a primary objective of the Army and Navy command. Asian flu in the '50s and Hong Kong flu in the '60s were ample warning that influenza could strike at any time.

In 1957 Purnell Choppin arrived at Rockefeller to join the Laboratory of Frank Horsfall and Igor Tamm, and just in time to confront Asian flu head on. Thus began his 29-year career at Rockefeller on influenza research. I was at Rockefeller with Maclyn McCarty and Rebecca Lancefield. Choppin and I had been house officers together at Barnes, remained friends, and I learned much from him then and later about flu and the prior contributions of Thomas Rivers, George Hirst, as well as Tamm and Horsfall, and their former colleagues including Edwin Kilbourne and Maurice Hilleman.

I recall the Asian flu of 1958 pandemic because several of my RHD patients were hospitalized at Rockefeller with influenza. They were high risk patients, extremely ill, and in heart failure, but survived. Did penicillin do the trick? Probably. I do not know for sure. The convalescent sera of several of these patients were used by Choppin for various studies on Asian influenza virus because they had unusually high titers of hemagglutinins.

This is a good time to introduce the discovery in 1945 by George Hirst of agglutination of RBC by flu virus. He was at Rockefeller, and Rebecca Lancefield remarked to me a decade later that Hirst's discovery was a major topic of conversation in the Welch Hall Dining Room where scientists from different laboratories lingered over a leisurely lunch to discuss recent research with colleagues in other laboratories. A significant consequence of these discussions on Hirst's discovery is recorded by Corner in his history of Rockefeller.[9]

"Hirst thought clumping of red blood cells by influenza viruses might depend upon the presence of polysaccharides on the cell surfaces. Hotchkiss suggested that he could test this supposition by treating the red blood cells with periodic acid, which destroys polysaccharides by converting them to new compounds (aldehydes). The idea proved correct; the treated cells would no longer agglutinate. Hotchkiss, aware that aldehydes form colored compounds with the well-known Schiff's reagent, next suggested that a staining method to reveal the presence of polysaccharides could be based on this sequence of reactions. Hotchkiss ' … showed this stained …' a wide variety of natural polysaccharides, leaving other tissue ingredients untinged … Walther Goebel used it successfully to demonstrate the oxidation of polysaccharides in dysentery bacilli. Since then it has been put to work in many biological investigations. Dermatologists have found that it sharply reveals the presence of fungi infecting the human skin, and the Hotchkiss stain is now in standard use for a practical purpose quite unforeseen by its inventor."

Choppin has recalled for me the early genetic evidence by George Hirst that suggested the influenza virus genome was in several pieces, in many ways, the most important discovery on influenza at Rockefeller after Francis' earlier contributions. Following the initial observations by Hirst in 1962,[10] subsequent studies by several investigators using sucrose gradient centrifugation and polyacrylamide gel electrophoresis revealed at least five distinct pieces of RNA; later eight were identified.

Between 1970–74, I was a member of the NIAID Infectious Disease Advisory Committee. Several times a year, we reviewed the various protocols for evaluation of vaccines including influenza that were conducted in the vaccine evaluation units then supported by NIAID. We were kept abreast of the efforts to match the flu strains incorporated into the vaccines with the anticipated wild strains that would circulate in the coming season. During these meetings I became aware of this important finding concerning influenza gene segments and the explanation they provide for the antigenic shifts seen earlier by Francis and others. This, of course, stems from the recognition that the genetic code for the hemaglutinin and the neurominadase are on different gene segments, and that the simultaneous infection of a single cell by two different flu viruses can lead to a re-assortment of the genes in the virus progeny. So I had been primed to this extent about the vagaries of influenza shift and drift at the time I became Director of NIAID in November 1975.

These reminiscences set the stage for my confrontation of the events surrounding what has come to be called "the swine flu affair," which occurred just six weeks after I became Director of NIAID. I had come from the Rockefeller University where, as I have said, I began laboratory research on streptococcal disease with Maclyn McCarty and Rebecca Lancefield. I arrived with a broad background in microbiology and immunology, with an interest in clinical medicine and clinical epidemiology. At the time that I was appointed Director, the microbiologists thought I was a microbiologist, and the immunologists thought I was an immunologist. Both groups were disappointed because during my time I supported both camps, and not one or the other. As I said at the time, and I still do, "infection and immunity are on opposite sides of the same coin."

In recalling the events concerning swine flu and for the preparation of these comments, I have *not* referred again to the book authored by Neustadt and Feinberg[11] entitled *The Swine Flu Affair: Decision-Making on a Slippery Disease*. So what follows is from memory, but I have prompted my memory by reading my oral history recorded in 1991 by Dr. Victoria Hardin in the NIH Office of Medical History, some of which I used in the Introduction of *Emerging Infectious Diseases* which I edited.[12]

Sometime during the first months of '76, influenza occurred at Fort Dix, New Jersey. There were several deaths and soon the Centers for Disease Control (CDC) and others determined that the cause was a swine flu virus, thought to be related to the virus that caused the pandemic of 1918. There were approximately 500 to 1000 young men infected in January and February as detected by conversion of serial sera from negative to positive for swine flu hemagglutinins. This was reported by Frank Top to the AFEB at the time. It was a mild disease except for one or two deaths. I recently learned from Dr. Donald Burke that he and his group have done a calculation of the reproduction rate from the available historical data, and it turns out to be $R_0 = 1.1 \sim 1.2$. This suggests that swine flu would not have become a major epidemic. We did not have those calculations at the time, nor were such calculations widely used. But as I told Dr. Burke, at least R_0 was >1, and not <1.

As you can imagine, in February 1976 meetings of the experts were called, and there was a general sense of alarm as well as a sense that something must be done to prevent an epidemic that might be a replay of 1918. All agreed that we needed to enhance US-wide and worldwide surveillance to determine the extent of a possible major outbreak of this virus. Should we prepare a vaccine as soon as possible with the swine flu virus, and immunize as much of the population as could be achieved by the following September so that children would be immunized by the time school convened? That was the question. In January and for the next ten months, there were frequent consultations on this matter with Dr. David Sencer, Director, CDC in the lead; and Dr. Harry Meyer, Director, BOB, and myself, Director, NIAID. Hovering over us with great care and attention was Dr. Theodore Cooper, Assistant Secretary for DHEW.[c] Hardworking backups to us included Dr. Hope Hopps, Bureau of the Biologics; Dr. Walter Dowdle, CDC; and Dr. John Seal, Deputy Director, NIAID. Later Dr. William Jordan and Dr. John LaMontagne joined the NIAID circle. Dr. Maurice Hilleman of Merck frequently joined an informal group for intense discussions on the clinical trials that were done in the spring of 1975 with the vaccines quickly prepared by the industry and a careful review of the antibody titers in the volunteers immunized with the vaccine. NIAID was supporting four centers for testing in volunteers candidate vaccines for various microbes, including influenza. The Rochester University Center was one of those that tested the swine flu vaccine. I note in a recent press release that the NIAID-supported Rochester Center has conducted a vaccine trial for the avian flu H5N1. Dr. Anthony Fauci commented on this successful immune response to this vaccine in the volunteers.

As I recall sometime in February 1975, a group of intramural and extramural flu scientists reached a near consensus that the Fort Dix swine flu was likely to be the source of an imminent pandemic of influenza, perhaps similar to 1918, because Ft. Dix flu had the antigenic characteristics of what was thought to be the 1918 flu. There was at least one notable exception to

---

[c]Later DHEW was changed to Department of Health and Human Services (DHHS), and with that I remarked, "Now to be known as the Department of H_2S." Mr. Califono was not amused. I never understood the reason for changing "Welfare" to "Human Services." Delegates to the Constitutional Convention argued and debated just what word to use for "welfare" in the phrase of the Preamble "to promote the general welfare." That is, of course, one of the most important functions of government. Unfortunately, welfare has come to mean a free handout for layabouts. Fortunately, a Department of Education took up the responsibility for E in DHEW, and for that John Adams can rest comfortably. He had argued for a section in the Constitution concerning education for everyone. That was voted down at the Convention, but he did write into the Massachusetts Convention an item on education for all of the citizens of Massachusetts.

this consensus who thought it possible but unlikely that the Fort Dix flu would be the origin of a pandemic. If I recall, he noted that a flu epidemic began like a cloudburst in the population where it first makes its appearance, for example, in a cluster of school children, as was the case of the Asian flu in 1958. Maurice Hilleman got a headstart on that epidemic by obtaining a number of flu samples collected from those Asian children who were among the first to be infected. Also I recall an occasion in March '76 when Donald Fredrickson, then the Director of NIH, and I were driving down to the Hubert Humphrey Building to brief Dr. Cooper on the plan to move ahead with vaccine production with the intent to immunize 50 million people. Don cautioned, "This thing is moving too fast." That was the gut feeling of a distinguished scientist in an entirely different field of research.

Throughout the spring and summer we monitored carefully for the occurrence of swine flu elsewhere in the world, and particularly in the Southern Hemisphere as the winter season was occurring there. There were scattered reports of an occasional case of swine flu in farmers in the Midwest. What to do? Should the vaccine be stockpiled? The argument against stockpiling the vaccine was a strong one. The vaccine had to be given before the putative epidemic occurred in September/October 1976, so it was a race against time. Yet, there were those who said wait and see. In the end the decision was made to go ahead.

After much consultation and discussion at the highest levels of the US Government, the Public Health Service launched a crash program to fund the commercial manufacture of sufficient swine flu vaccine to immunize 50 million people. This was achieved during voluntary mass immunization by October, ten months after the alarm was sounded. The epidemic did *not* occur, however.

So the Ft. Dix episode was a false alarm, and the public and much of the scientific community accused us of overreacting. As someone noted, it was the first time we have been blamed for an epidemic that did not occur.

It is worth noting that there is an upside to the swine flu episode. In some ways it was one big fire drill. We proved it was possible to organize a mass influenza immunization program from start to finish: identify the virus, grow up stocks, prepare and field test the vaccine, provide for indemnity, and immunize a large segment of the population, all within ten months. We learned a great deal from that drill, and I am sure we can do better the next time. The day will come when we will again retrace this race against time.

I have called the uncertainty that surrounds any response to a microbial outbreak the Fog of Epidemics, analogous to the Fog of War of which the historians speak.[12]

The Fog of War: Uncertainty
    Where is the enemy?
    What is his strength?
    What counterattack?
The Fog of Epidemics: Uncertainty
    Where is the microbe?
    How many; how virulent; how communicable?
    What counterattack?
Perceived Miscalculations
    1975 Swine flu outbreak
    Response too rapid
    1981 HIV/AIDS occurrence
    Response too slow

In the case of swine flu, we may have acted too soon. And in the case of AIDS, we may have acted too slowly. Read the book by Neustadt and Fineberg[11] for a full account of our perceived folly in regard to swine flu. For an account of the perception that between 1981–84, as Director of NIAID, I dithered and dithered over the onset of the HIV/AIDS epidemic, read what Shilts says about me in *And the Band Played On*.[13]

I relate these personal reminiscences because many who read this chapter will be on the firing line when future epidemics threaten, and they will either erupt or fizzle out. You will be in a fog, and you will need to exercise the best judgment you can on the basis of an assessment of the *surveillance* information, and the historical context. Roy Anderson and others have been on the firing line in the UK to advise on policies to contain bovine spongiform encephalopathy (BSE) in cattle and to curtail the possible transmission to humans, and later to advise on policies to limit the spread of foot and mouth disease. And now DHHS, CDC, NIAID, WHO and the MOH of many countries in Southeast Asia are on the firing line in regard to chicken flu. Stockpile drugs? Prepare a vaccine? Prepared a vaccine for chickens and use it now? Cull infected flocks now? What to do? No matter what you do when faced with difficult choices, you will be criticized. But as President Truman said, "If you can't stand the heat, stay out of the kitchen."

Any narrative on the swine flu episode would be incomplete without mention of the work of Richard Shope, also at Rockefeller, on the possible relationship between the putative influenza virus of 1918 and its eventful residence in pigs in Iowa where it caused an influenza-like syndrome and where it remained as a reservoir.[14]

Sir Christopher Andrews in his biographical memoir on Shope wrote as follows:[15]

"During 1937, sera were obtained from pigs at farms near two institutions where flu outbreaks were in progress: the results showed that the pigs too had become infected with the human viruses. These observations suggested that swine influenza, which had first been observed in the Midwest in 1918, might have originated *from the transmission of the pandemic virus from man to pig.* This idea was put forward independently by Laidlaw in Britain and by Shope. Remarkable confirmation came from studies of antibodies in people of different ages. Shope found, in 1936, that hardly any human sera from children aged 12 or less would neutralize the swine flu virus while many from older persons did so. This suggested that a virus antigenically related to swine flu had been present in the human population up to 1924 but not later. (One may reasonably suppose that the virus responsible for the 1918 pandemic persisted for a few years after that catastrophe.) Work in several laboratories has confirmed these suggestions and the relation of swine flu virus to the pandemic strain is generally accepted as being highly probable."

Whatever the merits of this argument about the cause of swine flu virus infection in adults in the 1930s, of interest here is Francis' suggestion that the swine flu antibody in humans was the result of repeated exposure to human strains, and perhaps not due to prior infection with the 1918 virus. Surely his thoughts about this matter were the genesis of his concepts expressed in "On the Doctrine of Original Antigenic Sin" published in 1960.[16] Francis wrote:

"The antibody of childhood is largely a response to dominant antigen of the virus causing the first Type A influenza infection of the lifetime. The antibody forming mechanisms are highly conditioned by the first stimulus so that later infections with strains of the same type successfully enhance the original antibody to maintain it at the highest level at all times in that age group. The imprint established by the original virus infection governs the antibody response thereafter. This we have called the Doctrine in the Original Antigenic Sin."

Thomas and Shope were very good friends. Shope spent his whole working life at Rockefeller and Francis, as was noted, was influenced by Shope and others to try his hand at influenza research. Yet in his 1953 paper[1] Francis was uncertain about the relationship between 1918 flu and swine flu.[1] He notes:

"The only significant suggestion is that the swine influenza virus is the 1918 strain, a proposal advanced originally by Laidlaw and by Shope. Antibodies to that virus are demonstrable in the serum of the human population. In 1936 Shope, and Andrewes, Laidlaw and Smith, observed that they were commonly found in persons over ten years of age but quite infrequently below that age. It was suggested that these antibodies were the result of specific infection with the 1918 virus which in 1935 was no longer prevalent in man but had become established in swine. On the other hand, swine virus is related to other strains of Type A influenza virus, and we had noted that repeated inoculations with the latter strains induced immunity and antibodies to the swine virus. *It seemed to us that, from this point of view, antibody to swine virus observed in man was instead the result of a broadened, composite antibody spectrum stimulated by repeated exposures to the related human strains.* In support of this concept are the repeated observations that persons recovering from identified infection with later Type A viruses may exhibit a rise in antibodies to swine virus, in some instances even in young children having their earliest experience with influenza virus, Type A. Whatever the answer, it is clear that strains having cross-relationship with swine virus have been prominent in human epidemics. Accordingly, if that virus represents the pandemic disease of 1918, it can be incorporated in vaccine. *Once again, however, I raise the question as to whether any single strain is the 'pandemic' strain, but with proper virulence, a variety of strains can produce the effect.*"

In his 1953 paper[1] Francis takes issue with the often stated view that the 20–35 age group had higher incidence and mortality than did other age groups during 1918 influenza. He writes:

"Nevertheless, the clinical behavior of that 90%–95% of illnesses which were uncomplicated, the major epidemiologic pattern and the evidence of immunity in the population seem to characterize it as influenza associated with a virus which had previously been in circulation. *The disagreement centers largely about the matter of age of incidence and of mortality, for which there are but limited data.*"

... He noted the "excessive and disproportionate incidence of pneumonic complications in the 25 to 40 age group of 1918. It has led to the common conclusion that influenza in that year more commonly affected persons of 25 to 40 ... The 25 to 40 age group had an intermediate incidence of influenza, the highest frequency of pneumonic complications and a high case fatality, although less than that in the later ages ... The incidence of infection does *not* indicate that the virus infection of 1918 selectively attacked the 25 to 40 group."

Francis died in 1969 and did not live to know the full explanation for virus antigenic shifts through the re-assortment of the gene segments of two parent viruses, or the antigenic drift through mutations. It will take additional research in the archives to know what speculations he made at the time on the matter of the genetics of antigenic shift, given the state of genetic knowledge about flu at the time of his death. He surely would have been in awe as we all are of the molecular explanation of flu virus variation with succeeding epidemics. And yet, even with the brilliant work of Taubenberger on the delineation of the 1918 virus, we can still ask Francis' question, is this "the pandemic strain" that can return again to haunt us? I believe he would be cautious about that. Yet, he surely would have agreed that knowledge about the genetics of the 1918 flu will guide us in the recognition of those characteristics of "the" future viruses that have "the proper virulence." And I believe he would be cautious also about the pandemic potential of the current chicken flu. Be prepared, yes. Keep alert to the unexpected. Be prepared for a *Newe Acquayantance*.

In 1968 Francis gave a brief talk at the First International Conference of Virology in Helsinki.[17] This was to be his last published work. His topic: "Moments in Medical Virology."

He mentioned three moments: First the discovery of bacterial viruses; second, Rous' report that rabbits kept for a long period after inoculation with the Shope papilloma virus had developed genuine cancers. The third was the transformation of the pneumococcus. He then goes on to relate his own early research on transformation when he first joined Avery's laboratory, and his efforts to extend Griffith's *in vivo* observations to *in vitro* experiments.

"So I spent the mornings in the laboratory learning of these phenomena and the afternoons in the library and on the tennis court developing a model of the double fault. Being convinced that the induced change of pneumococcus types in the animal host was a true bill, I began very primitive efforts to obtain transformation in the test tube. (It is worth noting that a healthy air of skepticism surrounded the entire phenomenon — that probably some live organisms were persisting in the heated, supposedly, killed preparation.) It became clear that the capsular polysaccharide, with all its divine properties, was not the effective agency. Then it seemed likely that whatever the transforming principle was, it needed special care and I began making extracts by freezing and thawing organisms in the cold under relatively anaerobic conditions so as to avoid an enzymatic destruction of the principle.

One day at noon I thought I was all alone in the lab. I was occupied with the tedious procedure of freezing and thawing. I had put my head down on my arms on the desk. Unexpectedly, a quiet voice said, 'What's the matter, boy?' Startled, I said I hated to see another pneumonia season start with the great time and attention required for clinical work; that I thought what was in these flasks was more exciting. Then I received a very sharp lecture from Dr. Avery reminding me that we were physicians; that the major concern of this laboratory was lobar pneumonia and that what was done here was in effect to understand the disease and to lick the pants off the pneumococcus — a theme that was developed under Avery and Dubos with the Type III decapsulating enzyme. This is a true view of Avery's intellectual commitment to the clinical problem.

New lines of effort were freely allowed even if they were not always enthusiastically supported. I found this when I studied transformation of the rough Type III to virulent in rabbits; there was a lot of specificity involved and much work, but it never was published until later (by others)... Things were apparently dormant for ten years.

Then came the epochal paper by Avery, MacLeod and McCarty in 1944 ..."

McCarty confirms that Francis actively worked in the field of transformation for a time.[18]

Francis makes no mention in these three moments in virology of his own large body of work on flu and polio. In recalling his early tentative research on transformation, was there a sense of regret that he had not stuck with it, and therefore he had missed out as an author on the paper that has been elevated to the centerpiece in the canon of molecular genetics? I think not. Anton Chekhov tells us that "the Turk digs a well so that he leaves behind something to be remembered." So be it with Tommy Francis. He dug a well. He dug deep. He will be remembered.

I met Francis on a number of occasions in the '50s and '60s. This came about in an indirect way. In 1950–51, I worked with Charles H. Rammelkamp (Rammel), Jr., and others including Floyd Denny, Lewis Wannamaker, and Chandler Stetson at Warren Air Force Base, Cheyenne, WY, on the initial studies that proved conclusively that penicillin treatment of streptococcal sore throat would prevent rheumatic fever (RF), and rheumatic heart disease (RHD). This research was supported by the Armed Forces Epidemiological Board (AFEB). Dr. Francis was active on various Commissions of the AFEB and I was affiliated at the time also with the Streptococcal Commission, and therefore met with Board members including Francis.

John Paul recalls in his memoir on Francis for the US National Academy of Sciences[5] that Francis "developed early in life the characteristic of combining seriousness with an excellent sense of humor" — That was very true. I remember a 1962 NIH conference on the etiology of primary atypical pneumonia. Was the microbe a virus, strep. MG, or the Eaton agent? What was it? Masur Auditorium was packed with pneumonia experts; John Dingle, Floyd Denny, Robert Austrian and many others. The bombshell at the conference was Bob Channock's report that the elusive Eaton agent was a mycoplasma. During the course of the discussions, Tommy Francis arose and remarked, "We have just heard what I call Peter Pan research, sometimes it *peters* out and sometimes it *pans* out!"

John Dingle closed the conference with the verdict that "Koch's postulates have been fulfilled."

Another occasion when I met Tommy Francis also has a humorous twist to it. Each spring, for many decades, there was a migration of clinical investigators from all over the country to Atlantic City to attend the three clinical research meetings — the "Young Squirts," the "Young Turks," and the "Old Turks," or the Association of American Physicians. On the last night, the Old Turks held a black-tie banquet, and after the banquet speaker, the Old Turks would parade up and down the boardwalk in their dinner jackets. Many gave off an air of importance, even if they were not. We, the Young Squirts, leaned against the boardwalk railing to gawk, perhaps even to do ourselves some good by hooking up with one or two of the Old Turks as they spilled out of Haddon Hall for a breath of fresh air. I joined Tommy Francis and Rammel, both in their tuxedos, and we walked some length down the boardwalk as far as the Brighton Hotel, where, on a previous evening by long tradition, one and all had gathered for Brighton punch, about as miserable a mixed drink as is the Singapore Sling.

On the way, Tommy Francis told us many stories about his years at Rockefeller and as the Chief Resident of the Hospital. I was at Rockefeller at the time, so I was all ears. Tommy was recounting events of 1933, a big time for him, because, as I have noted, his influenza research looked promising, and secondly he had just been married, and was about to take off for a honeymoon on the night sleeper to Niagara Falls. Suddenly, he had a call from Dr. Rufus Cole, the Hospital Director, informing him that a VIP needed medical attention. Such was one of the responsibilities of the Chief Resident, and, by tradition, all of the Rockefeller physicians. Many of these special patients were admitted to the Rockefeller Hospital. Francis was informed that the patient was a member of the Rockefeller family. When Tommy protested that he was about to take off on his honeymoon, Rufus Cole replied, "You must delay your departure. You are needed here!" A limousine was sent for him to make a house call on the patient, and a ticket was purchased for a night sleeper for a later day. So his wife went on to Niagara Falls without him. Thus it was that Tommy was late for his honeymoon.

Tommy recalled several other such stories about life at Rockefeller. By now it was at least 11 o'clock, if not later, and Tommy announced that he wanted a sandwich. We found a coffee shop off the boardwalk where he ordered "half a sandwich." This puzzled the counter man, but soon he delivered up half a sandwich. Rammel and I each had a coke.

I will not summarize this commentary, but close with the last paragraph of Francis' 1953 paper on "The Newe Acquayantance,"[1] and with his final comments in: "On the Doctrine of Original Antigenic Sin."[16]

"I have attempted to review the characteristics of the pandemic Disease of 1918 in the broad framework of our knowledge of influenza and influenza viruses. Although we are confronted with a changing population of new acquaintances, it is apparent that they represent a body of old associates varying in virulence and in antigenic characteristics. As the knowledge of their antigenic components increases, the probability that they can be countered by vaccine of proper composition improves, thus leading to the prevention and control of the last of the unconquered plagues of mankind.

Children represent the most susceptible members of the population, and probably the most important material for the building of epidemics. The gaps in their immunity should be eliminated by providing early in life the antigenic stimuli to meet the known or anticipated recurrent strains. Natural exposures would then serve to enhance the broad immunity laid down by vaccination. Could it

be that such vaccines can be made from pools of chemically purified antigens, or even with strains experimentally devised? In this
manner, the original sin of infection could be replaced by an initial
blessing of induced immunity."

Did Tommy Francis foresee the use of pools of monoclonal antibodies
(passive immunity) and recombinant vaccines (active immunity) to stem the
epidemic tide, even pandemic influenza?

Acknowledgments

An edited version of this chapter was previously published in the *Emerging
Infectious Diseases* Journal, Vol. 12, No. 1, pp. 40–43, 2006 (by the Centers for
Disease Control and Prevention, USA).

References

1. Francis T, Jr. Influenza: The *Newe* Acquayantance. *Ann Int Med* 1953;39:203–221.
2. Dochez AR, Avery OT, Lancefield RC. Studies on the biology of streptococcus.
   I. Antigenic relationships between strains of *Streptococcus haemolyticus*. *J Exp Med* 1919;30:179–213.
3a. Lancefield RC. The antigenic complex of *Streptococcus haemolyticus*. II. Chemical and immunological properties of the protein fractions. *J Exp Med* 1928;47:469–480.
3b. Lancefield RC. The antigenic complex of *Streptococcus haemolyticus*. III. Chemical and immunological properties of the species-specific substance. *J Exp Med* 1928;47:481–491.
4. MacLeod CM. Thomas Francis, Jr., 1900–1960. *Arch Environ Health* 1970;21:226–229.
5. Paul JR. Thomas Francis, Jr., July 15, 1900–October 1, 1969. *Nat Acad Sci Biogr Ser* 1974;44:57–91.
6. Francis T, Jr. Transmission of influenza by a filterable virus. *Science* 1934;80:457.
7. Stuart-Harris C. The Thomas Francis, Jr., Memorial Festschrift. *Arch Environ Health* 1970;21:225–474.
8. Francis T Jr., Salk JE, Pearson HE, *et al.* Protective effect of vaccination against induced influenza A. *Proc Soc Exp Biol Med* 1944;55:104.
9. Corner GW. *A History of the Rockefeller Institute 1901–1953 Origins and Growth.* The Rockefeller Institute Press, New York City, 1964, pp. 511–512.
10. Hirst GK. Genetic recombination with Newcastle disease virus, polioviruses and influenza. *Cold Spring Harbor Symp Quant Biol* 1962;97:303–306.

11. Neustadt RE, Fineberg HV. *The Swine Flu Affair: Decision-Making on a Slippery Disease*. US Department of Health, Education and Welfare, Washington, DC USA, 1978.

12. Krause RM. *Emerging Infections*. Introduction edited by Krause RM. Academic Press, New York, 1998, pp. 1–22.

13. Shilts R. *And the Band Played On: Politics, People, and the AIDS Epidemic*. St. Martin's Press, New York, USA, 1987.

14. Shope RE. The influenzas of swine and man. In: *The Harvey Lectures, 1935–1936*. The Harvey Society, New York, 1937, pp. 183–213.

15. Andrewes C. Richard Edwin Shope, December 23, 1901–October 2, 1966. *Nat Acad Sci Biogr Ser* 1979;50:353–375.

16. Francis T, Jr. On the doctrine of original antigenic sin. *Proc Am Philos Soc* 1960;104:572.

17. Francis T, Jr. Moments in medical virology. In: *International Virology* (ed.) Melnick JL. Proceedings of the First International Congress for Virology, S. Karger, A.G., Basel, Switzerland, 1968, p. 224.

18. McCarty M. *The Transforming Principle: Discovering that Genes are Made of DNA*. W. Norton & Co., New York, USA, 1985, pp. 81–82.